I0820322

Mélanie en Véganie

# ULTRA PROTEIN

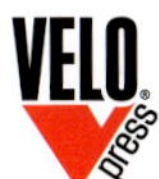

First printed in 2024 in France as *Ultra protéiné* by Hachette-Livre (La Plage).

Published in the US by:
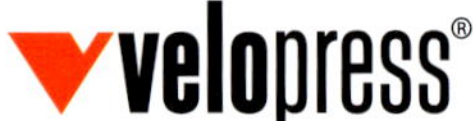

an imprint of Ulysses Press
32 Court Street, Suite 2109
Brooklyn, NY 11201
www.velopress.com

VeloPress is the leading publisher of books on sports for passionate and dedicated athletes around the world. Focused on cycling, triathlon, running, swimming, nutrition/diet, and more, VeloPress books help you achieve your goals and reach the top of your game.

ISBN: 978-1-64604-826-7
Library of Congress Control Number: 2025930801

Printed in India
10 9 8 7 6 5 4 3 2 1

Editorial direction: Céline Le Lamer
Editorial monitoring: Éléonore Doosterlinck
Graphic design: Nicolas Gallois
Proofreading: Charlotte Maillot
Layout: ZS studio
Production: Amélie Moncarré
Marketing and communications manager: Charlotte Couture
Partnerships Manager: Dana Lichiardopol

# SUMMARY



## INTRODUCTION



## SAVORY SNACKS



## SWEET SNACKS

## LUNCH



## DINNER

# THE ROLE OF PROTEINS

**Along with carbohydrates and fats, proteins are part of the macronutrients family. They are essential to our diet because they help our bodies develop and function properly.**

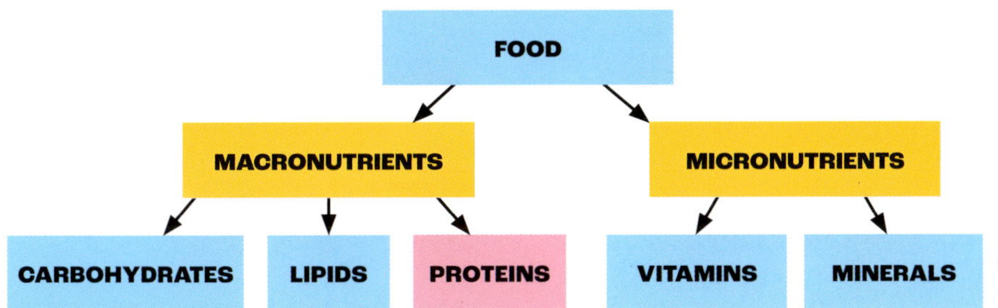


While carbohydrates and lipids primarily provide or store energy, proteins provide **the building materials** needed to form body structures. Thus, they are a primordial component of cells, organs, and even bones...

Proteins also play a role in many other bodily functions, such as blood clotting, the immune system, and the production of hormones and enzymes (among others!). You will soon understand these **macromolecules** are necessary for good health!

## PROTEIN CONSTRUCTION

To fully understand how they work, we need to analyze the molecules that proteins are composed of: **amino acids**.

Let's represent them visually: Amino acids are pearls that, once assembled, constitute a necklace. This would be a **protein chain**, also called **a polypeptide**.

A protein can comprise a combination of as few as 40 amino acid beads and up to nearly 30,000,[1] thus forming complex and functional molecular structures.

## THE DIFFERENT AMINO ACIDS

There are 20 different amino acids. Nine of them are said to **be essential**: They cannot be synthesized in the human body and must be provided by

---

**1** Valeri Barsegov, "Protein Primary Structure: Amino Acids," *University of Massachusetts Lowell,* February 14, 2019, http://faculty.uml.edu/vbarsegov/teaching/bioinformatics/lectures/ProtStructure1Modified.pdf.

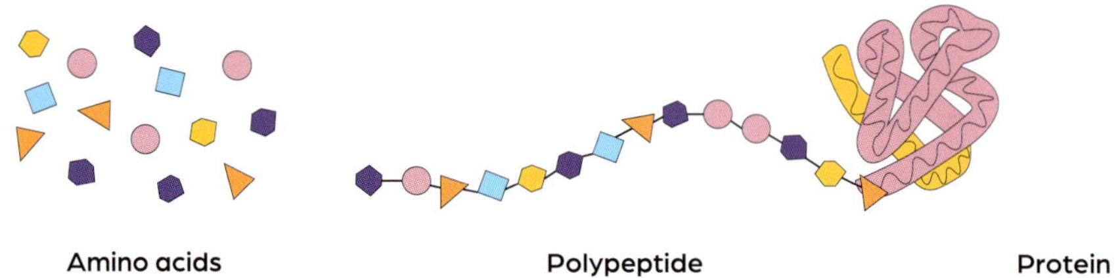


food: *histidine, isoleucine, leucine, lysine, methionine, phenylalanine, threonine, tryptophan,* and *valine*.

The other 11 are said to be **nonessential** and can be synthesized by the body from other components, even if they are not present in our diet: *alanine, arginine, asparagine, aspartic acid, cysteine, glutamic acid, glutamine, glycine, proline, serine,* and *tyrosine*.

With the exception of sugar and oils, all amino acids are present **in all foods**, whether animal or plant-based; they are simply present in varying quantities.

Eating only broccoli and peppers will not meet our protein quota but will still help absorb amino acids.

## THE DISTRIBUTION OF AMINO ACIDS

Professor Christopher Gardner, director of Stanford's Nutrition and Health program, uses an analogy from game Scrabble™ to understand the needs and distributions of amino acids: Certain letters like *e*, *m*, *a*, *o*, and *r* are common, while others like *z*, *y*, and *x* are rare. Amino acids work in the same way: Some, like tryptophan and cysteine, are rare simply because we have little need for them, while others, like glutamate and glutamine, are abundant because our bodies use them regularly!

For an intake of 40 g of protein, this doesn't mean that you need to absorb two g of each essential amino acid. You need **different amounts of each amino acid** to meet your body's needs.

You don't need protein as such but a good distribution of amino acids!

# AMINO ACID INTAKE BY FOOD GROUP[2]

All plant-based foods contain all 20 amino acids.

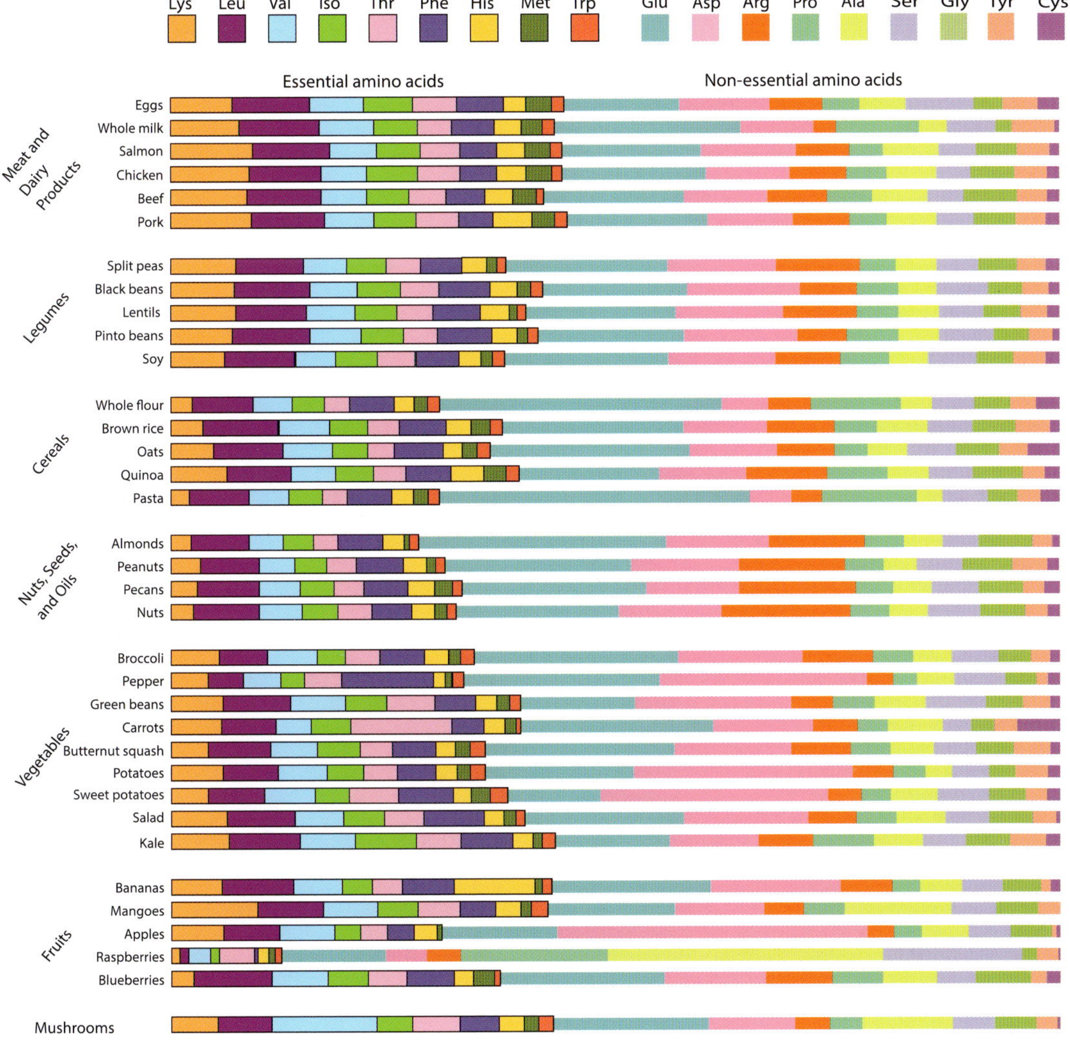


2 Christopher Gardner et al., "Maximizing the Intersection of Human Health and the Health of the Environment with Regard to the Amount and Type of Protein Produced and Consumed in the United States," *Nutrition Reviews* 77, no. 4 (2019): 197–215, https://doi.org/10.1093/nutrit/nuy073.

## "INCOMPLETE" PROTEINS AND AMINO ACID RESERVE

It is often said that animal proteins are "complete" and therefore superior to plant proteins, which are considered "incomplete." In fact, animal products provide an optimal distribution of the nine essential amino acids, while some plant protein sources, such as legumes and grains, are low in methionine and lysine, respectively. However, this does not mean that they are devoid of them. In theory, a diet consisting only of grains could lead to a lysine deficiency, but this problem is resolved when a varied diet is adopted. In practice, no one eats only grains. Furthermore, certain plants, such as soy, quinoa, or buckwheat, offer an amino acid distribution that is just as optimal as animal products. It is important to know that the body has a "reserve" of amino acids, which avoids having to consume all the essential amino acids in adequate quantities at each meal:[3] It is enough to regularly vary the sources of plant-based proteins from one meal to another to cover the body's needs. In practice, the notion of "incomplete" proteins thus loses its meaning because the body is capable of dealing with the different food intakes of the day.

# DAILY CONTRIBUTIONS

## CAN YOU EAT TOO MUCH PROTEIN?

In the US, we consume, across all diets, enough protein.[4] Although it is sometimes difficult to reach certain amounts of protein, there is no risk of deficiency.

Conversely, it isn't really known whether it can be dangerous to consume "too much" protein. Unlike lipids and carbohydrates, which have storage spaces in our bodies, there is no storage mechanism for proteins. Therefore, those consumed in excess of our functional needs are converted into carbohydrates and fats. As far as we know today, the threshold considered satisfactory is:

- minimum: 0.80 g/kg/day or 10% of the daily intake
- maximum: 2.2 g/kg/day or 27% of the daily intake

Some sources, including the United States Department of Agriculture (USDA)[5], estimate protein can be as high as 35% of the total energy intake (TEI).

---

[3] Food and Agriculture Organization of the United States et al.,"Protein and Amino Acid Requirements in Human Nutrition: Report of a Joint FAO/WHO/UNO Expert Consultation," *WHO Technical Report Series* 935, (2007), https://apps.who.int/iris/bitstream/handle/10665/43411/WHO_TRS_935_eng.pdf.

[4] Victor L. Fulgoni, "Current protein intake in America: Analysis of the National Health and Nutrition Examination Survey 2003-2004," *The American Journal of Clinical Nutrition* 87, no. 5 (2008): 1554S–57S–84, https://doi.org/10.1093/ajcn/87.5.1554S.

[5] USDA, "Dietary Guidelines for Americans 2020–2025," February 5, 2025, https://www.dietaryguidelines.gov/sites/default/files/2020-12/Dietary_Guidelines_for_Americans_2020-2025.pdf.

## LET'S DO THE MATH

The USDA considers that the recommended dietary allowance (RDA) for proteins for healthy adults varies based on age, sex, weight, and activity level. For males aged 19 and older the RDA average is **0.80 g/kg/day** or **56 g protein intake/day**. For women aged 19 and older the RDA recommends an average of **0.80 g/kg/day**, or **46 g protein intake/day**. The references of g of protein/day apply to **healthy sedentary adults**, but in many cases, it will be necessary to increase this dose. For example, **lactating women** are estimated to need 1.05 g/kg/day. An example of a lactating woman who weighs 65 kg (145 lbs) with regular physical activity: 1.05 g x 65 kg = 68.25 g protein per day.

BREAKFAST
LUNCH
SNACK
DINNER
English muffin with scrambled tofu
Spring rolls with tempeh
Carrot cake oatmeal
Caramelized TSP with sautéed vegetables
TOTAL
14 g + 28 g + 15 g + 17 g = 74 g

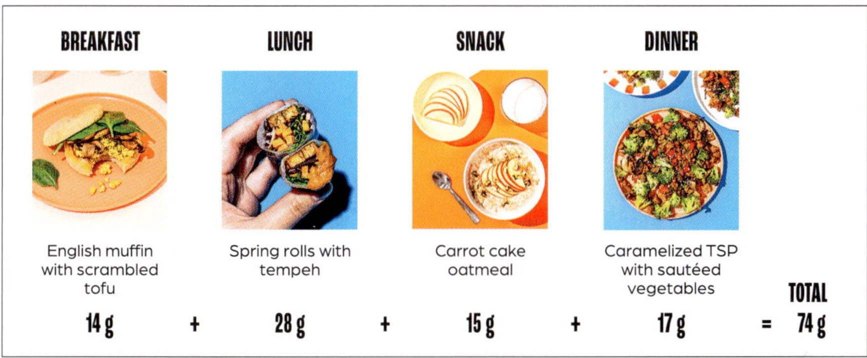

For a healthy adult, it is estimated that, on average, the caloric intake should be between 2,000 and 2,700 calories per day.

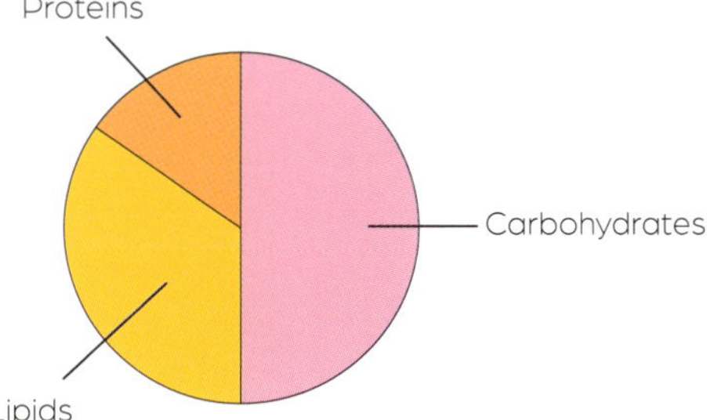


**Carbohydrates:** 40 to 55% of TEI
**Lipids:** 35 to 40% of TEI
**Protein:** 10 to 20% of TEI

# THE CONTENT IN PROTEINS

**Foods considered "high in protein" are those that allow us to meet our daily needs without exceeding our caloric intake, while taking into account our satiety, or the feeling of being full.**

## FOODS RICH IN PROTEIN

In Europe, a food is considered a source of **protein** if it contains at least 12% of calories from protein and **high in protein** if it contains at least 20% of calories from protein.[6] This means that a food is often considered high in protein if it includes around **5 g of protein or more per 100 g serving**.

Look at the table below: Many plant-based foods exceed this level and are considered "high in protein," but some are more strategic than others (see page 10).

## COMPARISON OF PROTEIN CONTENT PER 100 G[7]

| | | | |
|---|---|---|---|
| Spirulina | **60 g** | Tempeh | **17 g** |
| Nutritional yeast | **48 g** | Green beans | **16 g** |
| Lupin beans | **36 g** | Tofu | **14 g** |
| Chicken | **29 g** | Oats | **13 g** |
| Seitan | **29 g** | Egg | **13 g** |
| Flax seeds | **23 g** | Buckwheat | **12 g** |
| Peanuts | **23 g** | Lentils | **10 g** |
| Beef | **20 g** | Red beans | **9 g** |
| Chia seeds | **19 g** | Chickpeas | **8 g** |

[6] "Nutrition Claims," European Commission, March 18, 2025, https://food.ec.europa.eu/food-safety/labelling-and-nutrition/nutrition-and-health-claims/nutrition-claims_en.
[7] "Ciqual: French Food Composition Table," ANSES, February 2, 2025, https://ciqual.anses.fr/.

# STRATEGIC PLANT PROTEINS

**When you want to optimize your intake of vegetable proteins for sports, healing, because you are pregnant, or to rebalance your weight, it can be difficult to go above 70 g of protein per day. . . .**

## SATIETY AND PROTEIN INTAKE

Plant-based proteins are a source of **fiber**, which **affects our satiety**: We cannot consume 500 g of lentils for an intake of 50 g of protein because satiety will have taken effect before then. Furthermore, when you are trying to control your carbohydrate intake, you should know that plant-based proteins, such as whole grains or legumes, are also **sources of carbohydrates**, which can slow down weight loss, among other things. This is where—what I call—**strategic plant-based proteins** come in—those that most closely match the nutritional profile of meat: Lots of protein, few carbohydrates, and little fiber.

## TOFU, TEMPEH, SEITAN, TVP, IMITATIONS . . .

The protein content we are looking to obtain is at least 15 g per 100 g. That means with 150 g of tofu, we already ensure 22.5 g of protein, approximately double that of a portion of lentils of the same weight. This does not mean that you should not eat lentils. After all, they contain a very interesting nutritional package (a source of iron in particular); And integrating 150 or 200 g of one of these strategic proteins into a meal **effectively increases protein intake**.

Unless you are a high-level athlete whose diet directly impacts performance, there is no point in stressing about your protein intake. If one day you do not reach the quota, it will not change anything. You need to analyze your eating habits over entire weeks, not by looking at a single meal that was not nutritionally perfect.

***Pay attention to the values displayed***

***We sometimes read that legumes contain 20 to 25 g of protein per 100 g, but this is only true for their dry version! Once cooked, this rate decreases: They actually contain around 8 to 10 g of proteins per 100 g. If you have any doubts about the distribution of macronutrients in a food, you can check out this database: https://ciqual.anses.fr/.***

# A BALANCED PLATE

**From a purely nutritional point of view, there will never be a better recipe than simply putting the right proportions of whole foods on our plate.**

In a modern, healthy approach to eating, one of the key aspects is to focus on "protein" rather than "meat" by including various sources of plant-based protein.[8]

## FOOD GROUPS AND PROPORTIONS

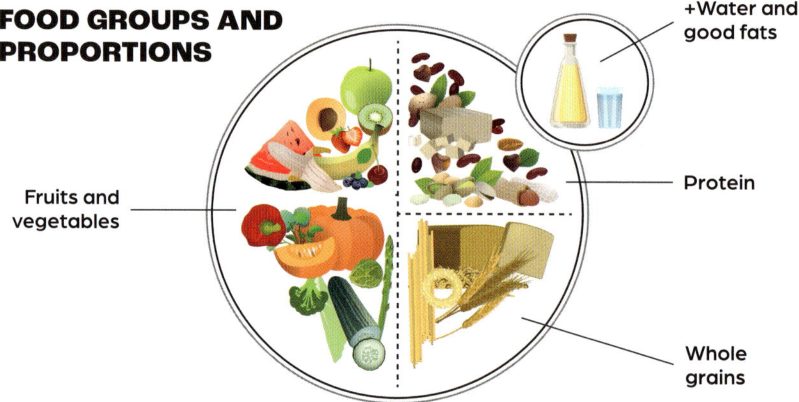


- **50% of fruits and vegetables:** This abundance of plants provides an effective source of vitamins, minerals, and fibers essential for good health. Salad, raw vegetables, stir-fried vegetables, oven-roasted vegetables with spices . . .
- **25% of whole grains:** Brown rice, quinoa, oats, and whole grain bread. They provide complex carbohydrates, fiber, and protein contributing to healthy digestion and stable energy levels throughout the day. Combining these sugars with fiber will help you avoid glucose spikes.
- **25% of protein:** Think about strategic plant-based proteins like tofu, tempeh, seitan, imitations, or textured vegetable proteins. Note to optimize your plate: I tend to put legumes with grains as they can also constitute your protein intake.
- When it comes to drinks, **water** is obviously recommended as the preferred choice: It supports all the essential bodily functions and it hydrates without calories or sugar.

**8** Recommended by Harvard's "Healthy Eating Plate" and Canada's food guide

## QUANTITY OF PROTEIN PER 100 G OF FOOD

**Tofu:** 15 to 18 g

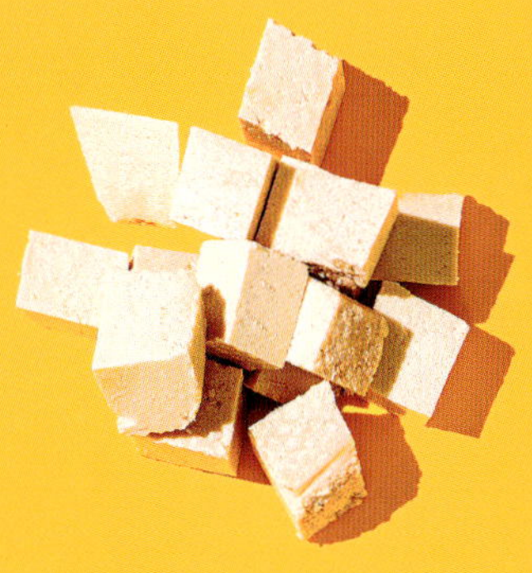

**Textured vegetable protein, textured soya protein (TVP, TSP):** 20 to 25 g

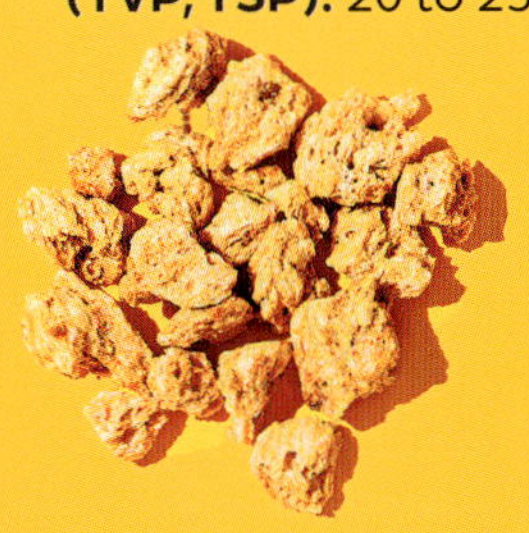

**Tempeh:** 15 to 20 g

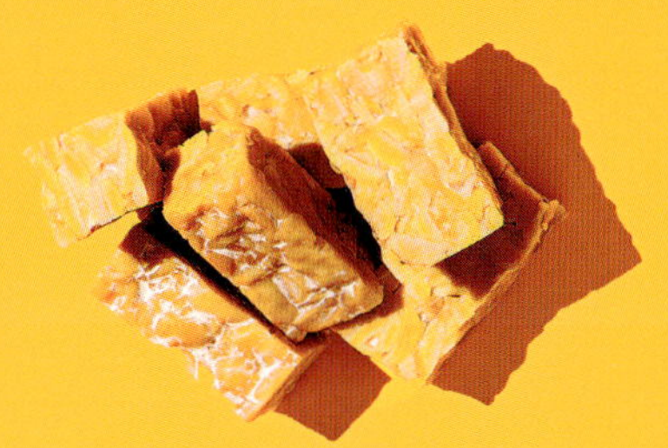

**Imitations:** 12 to 20 g

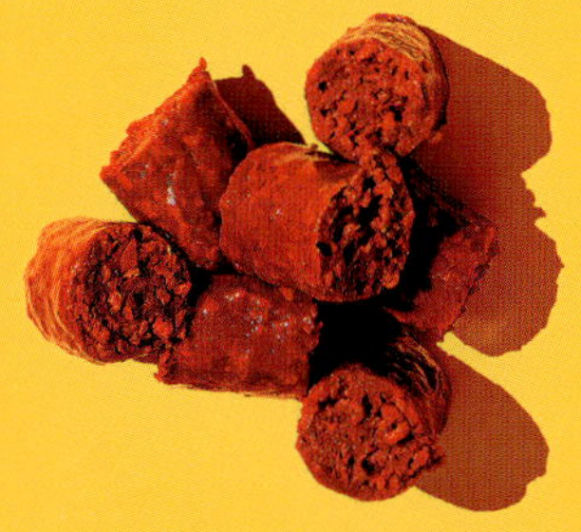

**Legumes:** 7 to 10 g

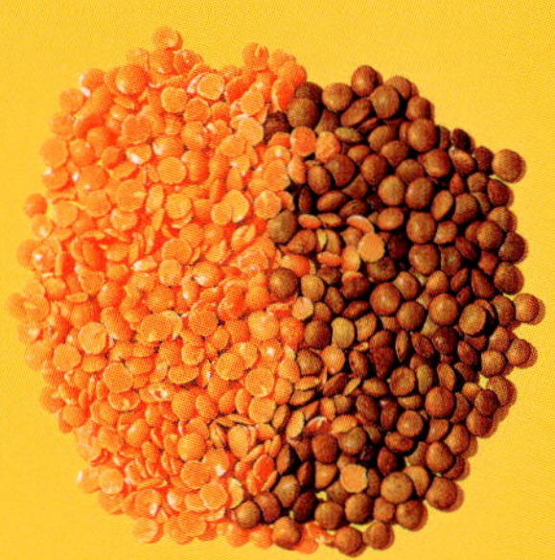

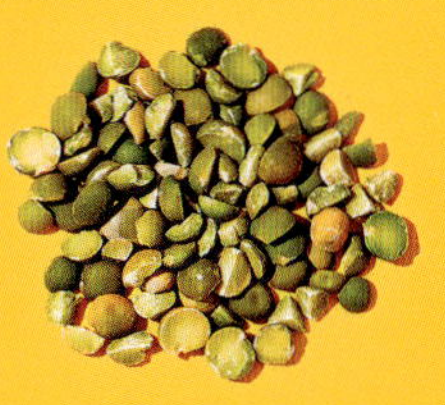

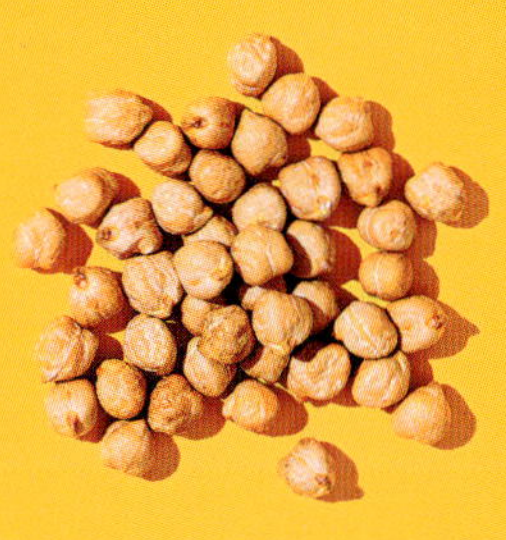

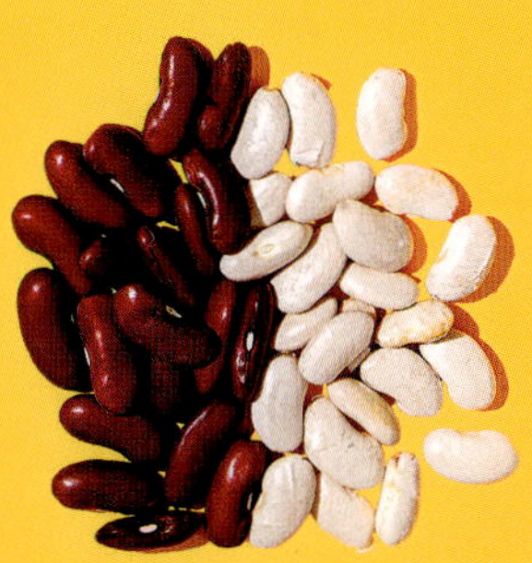

And 20 to 30 g for **seitan**!

**Whole grains:** 7 to 10 g
**Nuts:** 20 to 25 g
**Seeds:** 20 to 25 g
**Malted yeast:** 40 to 50 g

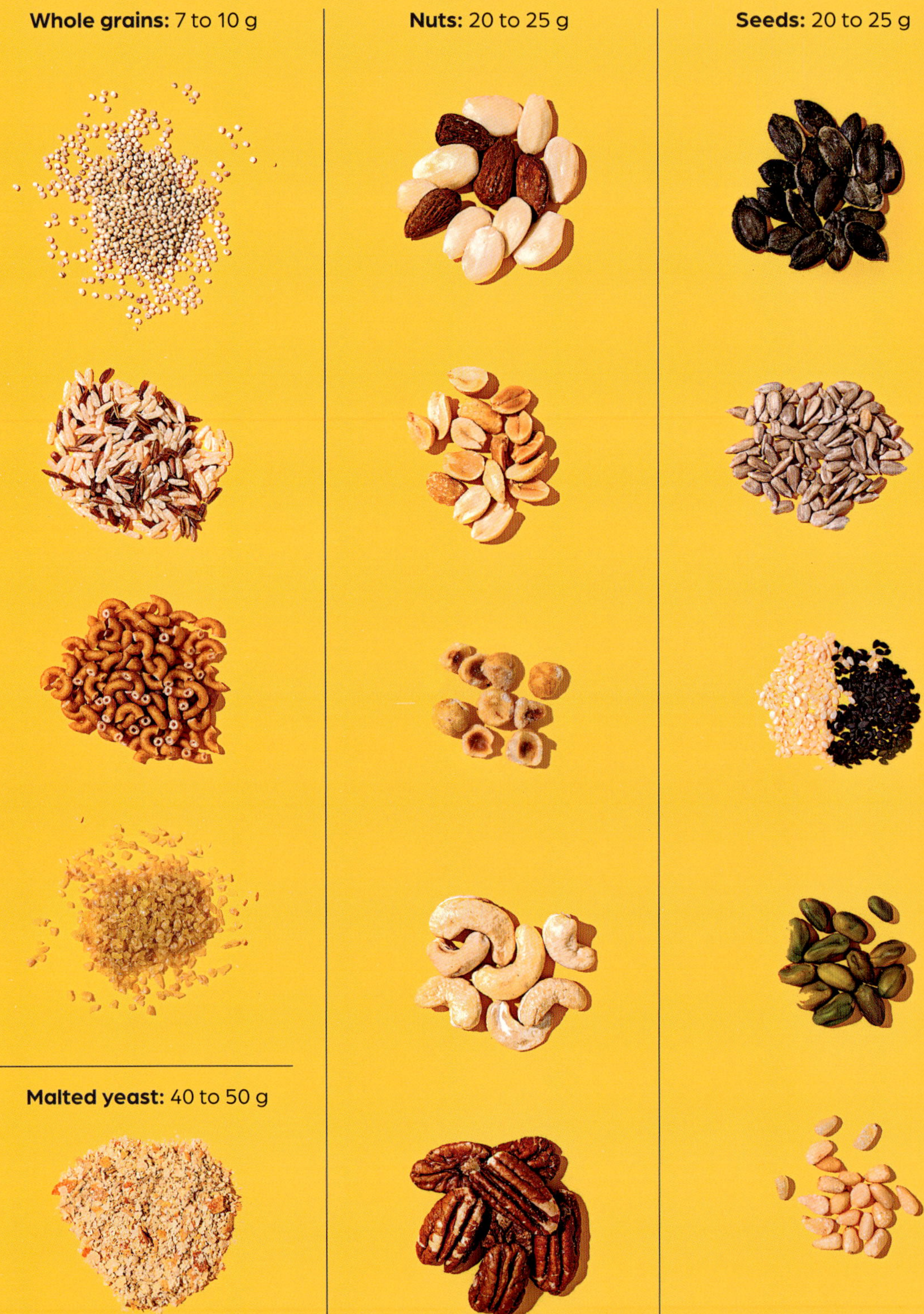

But also 60 g for **spirulina**, 20 to 30 g for **seaweed**, or 15 to 20 g for **hemp** . . .

# BOOST YOUR PLATES

**To easily increase your protein intake, there are a few food hacks that allow you to add a few grams here and there with minimal effort.**

| The hack | How to use? | Amount of protein |
|---|---|---|
| Nutritional yeast | Sprinkle on anything | 1 tablespoon = 4 g protein |
| Spirulina | Incorporate into smoothies or yogurts | 1 tablespoon = 4 g protein |
| Seeds: Pumpkin, sunflower, pine nuts . . . | Add to salads or pasta dishes | 1 tablespoon = 3 g protein |
| Nut butter: Almond, cashew, peanut . . . | Use in sauces and dressings | 1 tablespoon = 3 g protein |
| Tahini | Use in sauces and dressings | 1 tablespoon = 2 g protein |
| Ground flax seeds (to absorb omega-3) | Sprinkle on anything, incorporate into pastries | 1 tablespoon = 2 g protein |

### TIPS FOR INCORPORATING THESE FOODS INTO YOUR DAILY LIFE

- Buy them at organic stores or online grocery stores. To manage your budget, think about buying large quantities that you will keep for a long time or making your own nut butter with a blender, among other things. There is no need to buy everything at once; spread out your purchases if necessary.
- Keep them handy in jars or a drawer near your kitchen area for regular use.
- Establish routines:
  - In the morning, add spirulina to your yogurt.
  - For lunch, make a dressing with cashew butter for your salad, and sprinkle it with nutritional yeast and pumpkin seeds.
  - For a snack, add flax seeds to your smoothie.
  - For dinner, add nutritional yeast to your soup or pasta dish.

By following these tips, you can easily increase your daily intake of plant-based protein significantly. **It is the cumulative addition of these foods that has an impact.** With these additions, you can expect to get around 20 g of extra protein per day while diversifying your nutrient sources and making your meals tastier.

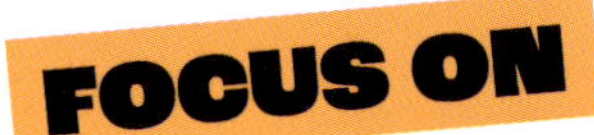


# PROTEIN POWDERS

## IN THE DAILY LIFE OF VEGETARIANS AND VEGANS

**Protein powders make your life easier on** days when you don't feel like cooking or when you haven't had time to get groceries.

**However, it is always best to get your nutrients naturally.** Whole foods provide essential fiber, vitamins, and minerals that powders can't replace; use protein powder as a supplement.

## AS PART OF EXERCISING

Protein supplements are commonly consumed by professional and recreational athletes, although purchase is often based on marketing claims rather than evidence-based research.

"Consuming protein powder can be an asset for athletes, but their effectiveness depends on the context. Taking a protein shake just before a physical effort does not have immediate effects if it is not part of a regular workout plan."[9]

In the long term, daily supplementation combined with suitable, frequent, and intense workouts can really boost your gain in muscle mass and strength. On the contrary, from a certain threshold, increasing protein intake no longer has any effect on muscle mass gain:[10] With above 1.6 g of protein/kg/day, athletes will not increase their muscle mass further. It is the stimulation of the muscle that makes it grow rather than the consumption of protein. For amateur athletes, without a structured program or with sessions that are too short, the effects are almost invisible. **The more protein you eat, the less powder you need.**

---

**9** Stefan M. Pasiakos et al., "Effects of Protein Supplements on Muscle Damage, Soreness and Recovery of Muscle Function and Physical Performance: A Systematic Review," *Sports Medicine* 44, no. 5 (2014): 655–70, https://doi.org/10.1007/s40279-013-0137-7.

**10** Robert W. Morton et al., "A Systematic Review, Meta-Analysis and Meta-Regression of the Effect of Protein Supplementation on Resistance Training-Induces Gains in Muscle Mass and Strength in Healthy Adults," *British Journal of Sports Medicine* 52, no. 6 (2018): 376–84, https://doi.org/10.1136/bjsports-2017-097608.

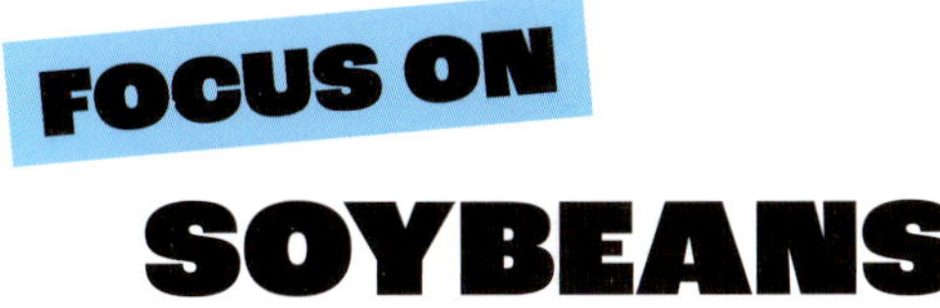


# SOYBEANS

**This nutritionally rich and absolutely versatile plant is the ideal alternative to many animal products.**

## A HEALTHY FOOD CONSUMED ALL OVER THE GLOBE

Consumed for over 3,000 years in Southeast Asia, soy is a food with a great deal of history. There is no evidence that its consumption has been linked to any kind of disorder. In Western countries, **this plant has also been adopted:** The United States affirms that pregnant and breastfeeding women and women suffering from breast cancer can consume soy; Canada recommends consuming it regularly as part of a varied diet; Australia recommends it as part of dietary diversification; and the United Kingdom has agreed to describe it as a healthy food.

| American Institute for Cancer Research | European Food Safety Authority (EFSA) |
|---|---|
| • No risk for people who have had breast cancer (even potentially reduces the risk of recurrence).<br>• No increase in prostate cancer.<br>• No risk but no specific interest in terms of prevention. | • Safe and appropriate for infant formula.<br>• No increased cancer risk.<br>• No change in thyroid hormones.<br>• No concerns about bone growth/health.<br>• No feminization or precocious puberty in children.<br>• Potential benefits for hormone-dependent cancers in adulthood.<br>• Included in a balanced diet. |

In France, an old report from 2005 written by AFFSA (formerly ANSES) issued precautionary principles due to interpretation difficulties and because results from experiments were carried out on animals. This is like being advised not to eat chocolate because dogs can die from it. It doesn't make sense! The only slightly controversial thing about soy is the isoflavones.

## ISOFLAVONE AND ESTRADIOL: SIMILAR STRUCTURE, DIFFERENT EFFECT

Soy has a high level of isoflavones, which are part of the phytoestrogen family of molecules found in plants. These isoflavone molecules have a structural resemblance to the female sex hormone: Estradiol. This similarity allows them to bind to estrogen receptors. Rather than being worrisome, this ability results in a modulation of estrogen receptors that **may be beneficial to health and may help balance hormonal effects:** Potential benefits could be managing menopausal symptoms and preventing certain cancers and cardiovascular risks.

At present, ANSES remains cautious and recommends not exceeding 1 mg of isoflavone/kg of body weight/day. When you calculate these precautionary measures, you can still consume one to two soy products per day. There is no data beyond a consumption of four portions per day, a threshold up to which no risk has been observed, but in any case, exceeding this limit would go against a varied diet and **does not materialize in real life**.

## IS SOY AN ENDOCRINE DISRUPTOR?

The second French national strategy on endocrine disruptors aims to identify and assess endocrine disruptors with the aim of reducing risks linked to chemical substances.[11] In this context, ANSES has listed 906 substances of interest, including 16 priorities, while the main isoflavones in soy (daidzein and genistein) are classified as category II, "unproven endocrine disruptors".

## WHAT ABOUT THE ENVIRONMENT?

Vegetarians and vegans are said to be causing deforestation in the Amazon rainforest due to all the soy they are eating: This is false! In fact, 77% of the world's soybeans are fed to livestock for meat and dairy production.[12] The remainder is used largely for biofuels, industry, or vegetable oils. Only 7% of soybeans are used directly to make human food products, such as tofu, soy milk, edamame beans, and tempeh. Look at the labels in supermarkets: **Soy is often organic and GMO free.**

---

**11** La deuxième stratégie nationale sur les perturbateurs endocriniens 2019–2022 (SNPE 2 2019–2022) [The second French national strategy on endocrine disruptors 2019–2020], https://www.ecologie.gouv.fr/sites/default/files/publications/SNPE%202%20english%20-%20Strategic%20objectives.pdf.
**12** Hannah Ritchie, "Drivers of Deforestation," *Our World in Data*, February 2021, https://ourworldindata.org/drivers-of-deforestation#is-our-appetite-for-soy-driving-deforestation-in-the-amazon.

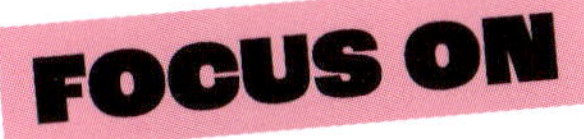


# IMITATIONS

As an innovative and practical solution for eating more plant-based foods, these alternatives have a good carbohydrate/protein ratio and offer interesting nutritional benefits. Some recipes are made with just soy, water, spices, and vitamin B12, offering a **healthy and simple option**. But not all products are equal, some imitations of red meat can contain less pleasant ingredients like methylcellulose (a food additive used to thicken and stabilize). Many vegan products still display a **Nutri-Score A**, guaranteeing acceptable nutritional quality!

## "IMITATIONS ARE PROCESSED PRODUCTS"

| Plant-based "bacon" | | Animal-based bacon |
|---|---|---|
| Rehydrated soy protein (82%), sunflower oil, salt, natural flavor, colorings: anthocyanin, lycopene; acidity regulator: potassium acetate. |  | Pork belly, preservatives: potassium lactate, potassium acetate, sodium nitrite; salt, dextrose, potassium chloride; antioxidant: sodium erythorbate. |

Plant-based alternatives do not necessarily have a longer ingredient list than animal products. For the former, the notion of processed food creates controversy; for the latter, it is accepted, and we even forget that animal products are processed products.

However, according to the WHO,[13] "there is sufficient evidence of the carcinogenicity in humans" of processed meats, and "approximately 34,000 cancer deaths per year worldwide are attributable to a diet rich in processed meats," states the Global Burden of Disease study[14].

---

**13** World Health Organization (WHO), https://www.who.int/en/news-room/questions-and-answers/item/cancer-carcinogenicity-of-the-consumption-of-red-meat-and-processed-meat (see "Processed Meat Was Classified as Group 1, Carcinogenic to Humans. What Does This Mean?'").

**14** World Health Organization (WHO), https://www.who.int/en/news-room/questions-and-answers/item/cancer-carcinogenicity-of-the-consumption-of-red-meat-and-processed-meat (see "How Many Cancer Cases Every Year Can Be Attributed to Consumption of Processed Meat and Red Meat?").

## PROMOTE SHORT INGREDIENT LISTS

In 2017, an American study highlighted that a vegetarian diet containing a significant quantity of ultra-processed products could lose its beneficial effects (in particular, protection against coronary heart disease) because they are often too salty, too fatty, and have too high of an energy intake.[15] Choosing products with a short ingredient list is a good way to consume good quality imitations.

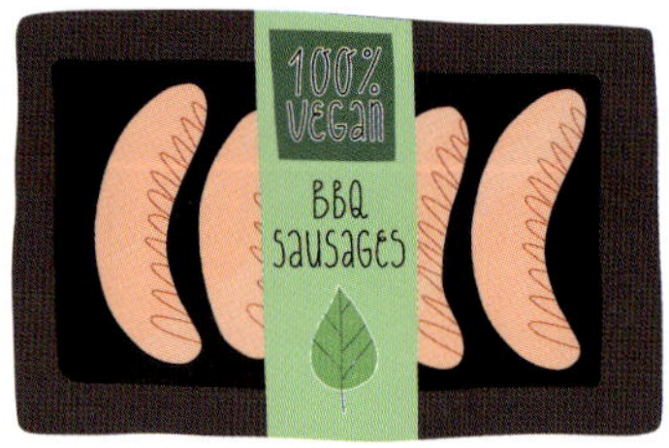


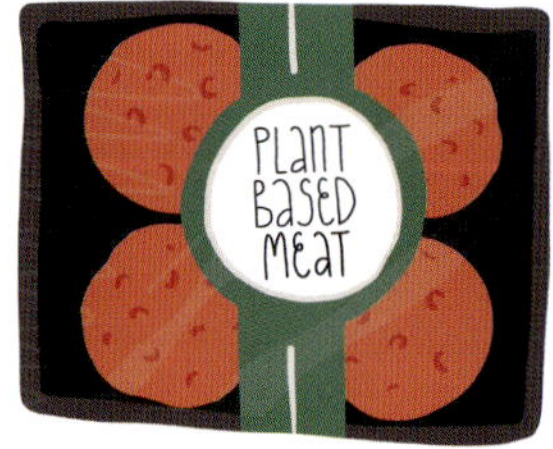


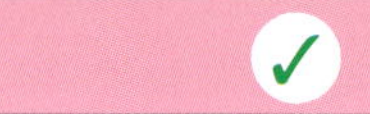

| ✓ | | ✗ |
|---|---|---|
| Water, pea protein (33%), pea fibre, rapeseed oil, vitamin $B_{12}$. | **VS** | Water, pea protein (16%), rapeseed oil, coconut oil, rice protein, flavoring, stabilizer (methylcellulose), potato starch, apple extract, color (beetroot), maltodextrin, pomegranate extract, salt, potassium chloride, concentrated lemon juice, corn vinegar, carrot powder, emulsifier (sunflower lecithin). |

A ratio of 80% of unprocessed foods and 20% of processed products allows you to enjoy these products while maintaining a nutritional balance. Consume them in moderation!

**15** Ambika Satija et al., "Healthful and Unhealthful Plant-Based Diets and the Risk of Coronary Heart Disease in U.S. Adults," *Journal of the American College of Cardiology* 25, no. 4 (2017): 411–22, https://doi.org/10.1016/j.jacc.2017.05.047.

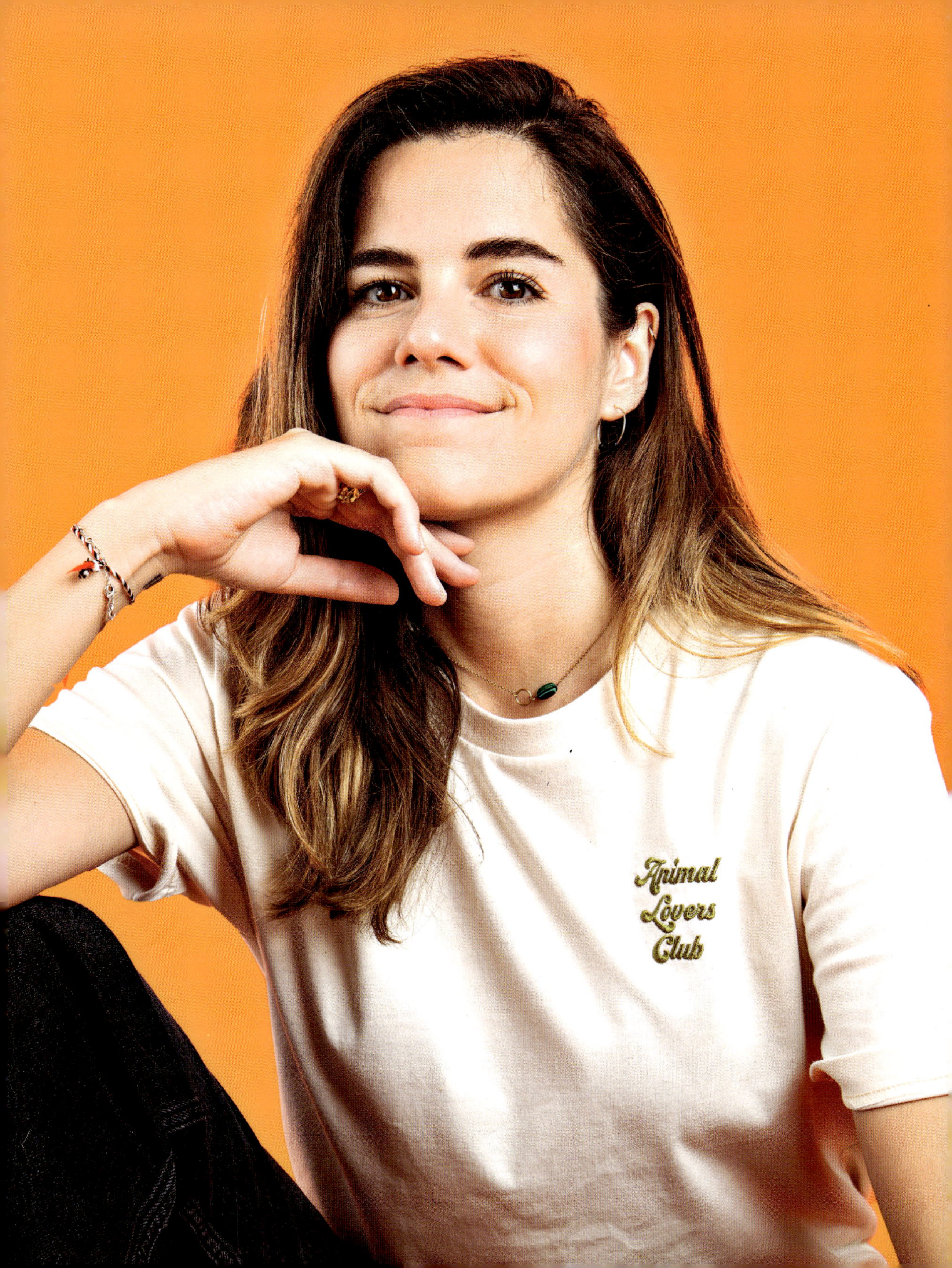
Animal
Lovers
Club

# INSTRUCTIONS FOR USE

This book allows you to explore plant-based proteins. I took care to highlight a wide variety of players: from the sometimes unpopular tofu, to the chickpeas that everyone knows, including chia seeds, cashew butter, nutritional yeast, tempeh, split peas, red lentil pasta, protein powder, or vegan bacon. . .

Despite an "ultra" enticing title, not all recipes are designed to deliver the maximum daily protein quota in a single meal. I would like to invite you to consider certain recipes as an integral part of a more complete meal to which you will need to add a starter and a side dish, as is the case, for example, with the quiche, which will "only" provide 10 g of protein per portion, but which should not be the only element on the plate. It is also necessary to compare like with like: A panna cotta intended to end the meal on a sweet note will not have the same nutritional profile as a double smash burger with red bean seitan, and that is completely normal!

Finally, is it possible to combine taste pleasure and nutritional optimization? I have tried to combine the best of both worlds, but it does not come without compromise. Cooking, simmering, gratinating, browning, frying: This provides satisfying flavors in the mouth but will sometimes "dilute" the protein content of a meal. Blending is still the best solution if you want to eat only nutrients. But this book also seeks to please our taste buds, which is an essential element for adopting plant-based proteins in the long term and learning to enjoy them!

Therefore, you will find many delicious everyday recipes, optimized with a maximum of protein sources and with correct-but-classic intakes, and ULTRA protein recipes that can exceed 40 g/portion to change the narrative and prove that it is possible! It's up to you to choose according to your needs.

This book is here to help you make informed and independent decisions about your food choices. Switching to plant based was the best decision I ever made! Enjoy eating and exploring!

**Mélanie**

# SAVORY SNACKS

- FOR 4 PEOPLE
- PREP/COOK TIME: 45 MIN
- REST TIME: 10 MIN
- ALL SEASONS

# SALTY BUCKWHEAT WAFFLES WITH TAHINI SAUCE

**FOR THE WAFFLES**

1½ cups (200 grams) **buckwheat flour**
2 tablespoons **cornstarch**
1 teaspoon **baking powder**
1 teaspoon **salt**
1¼ cups (300 milliliters) **soy milk**
2 tablespoons **olive oil**

**FOR THE TOPPING**

1 tablespoon **olive oil**
3½ ounces (100 grams) white **mushrooms**, sliced
3½ ounces (100 grams) **sun-dried tomatoes**
3½ ounces (100 grams) **arugula**

**FOR THE TAHINI SAUCE**

3 tablespoons **tahini**
**juice of ½ lemon**
1 **clove garlic**, minced
**salt** and **pepper**, to taste
some **water**, as needed

**1.** In a large bowl, mix the buckwheat flour, cornstarch, baking powder, and salt. Gradually add the soy milk and olive oil to the dry mixture, stirring well to avoid lumps. The dough should be smooth and consistent.

**2.** Let the dough rest for a few minutes while you prepare the topping and sauce.

**3.** Heat a skillet over medium heat with some olive oil. Sauté the white mushrooms until golden brown and tender. Reserve.

**4.** Make the tahini sauce by mixing the tahini, lemon juice, minced garlic, salt, and pepper in a small bowl. Adjust the consistency by adding a little water, according to your preference.

**5.** Heat a waffle iron. Then pour a portion of the batter into each mold and close it. Let the waffles cook until golden brown and crispy.

**6.** While the waffles are cooking, cut the sun-dried tomatoes into pieces.

**7.** Once the waffles are cooked, arrange them on plates. Top with the arugula, sun-dried tomatoes, and sautéed white mushrooms. Drizzle generously with tahini sauce.

## Tip

If you don't have a waffle iron, you can turn the waffles into savory pancakes using the same batter.

FOR 100 G

| protein: **6.7 g** | carbohydrates: **28.4 g** | lipids: **10.6 g** |
|---|---|---|

PER SERVING (230 G)

| protein: **13.4 g** | carbohydrates: **56.9 g** | lipids: **21.2 g** |
|---|---|---|

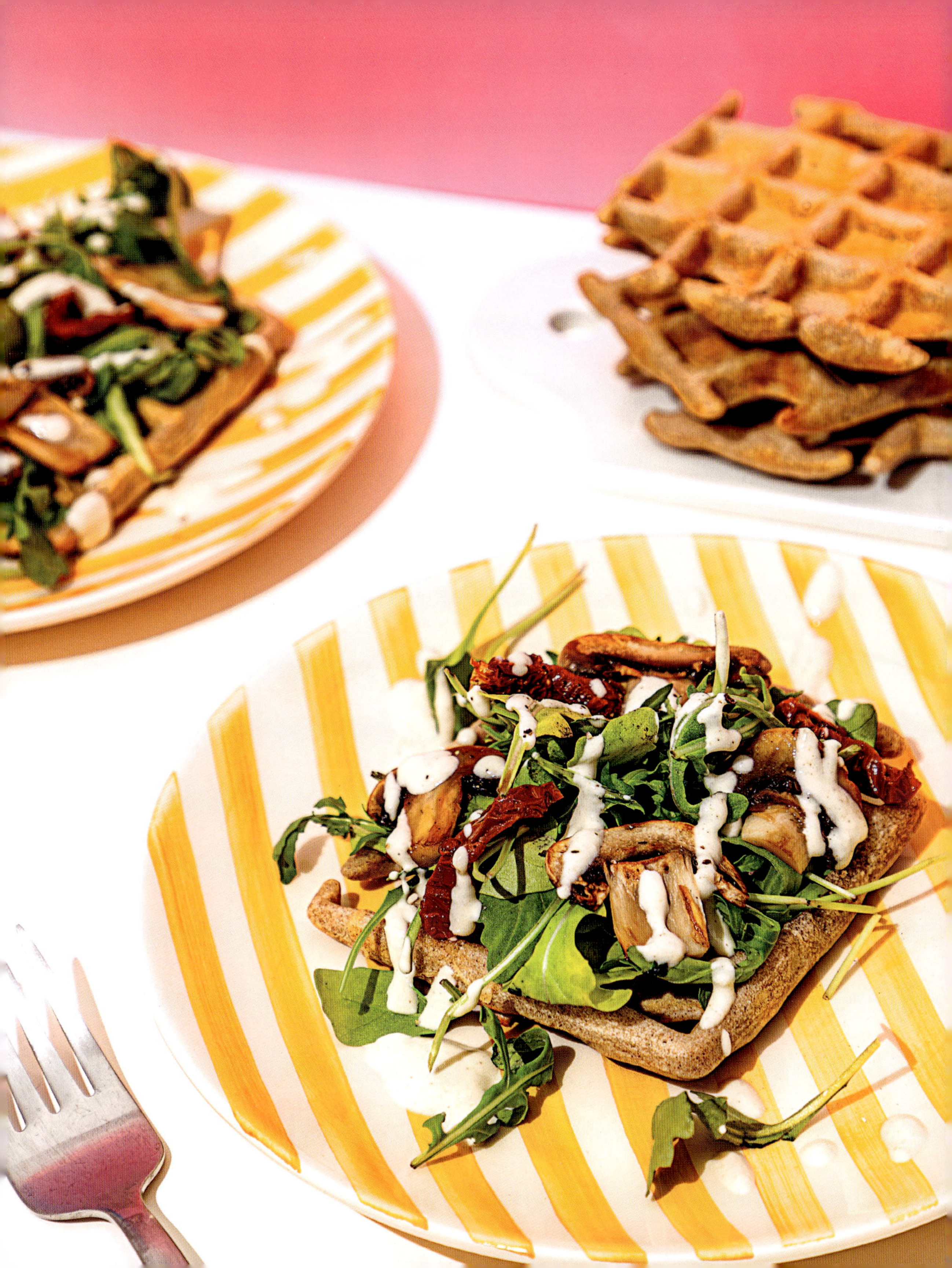

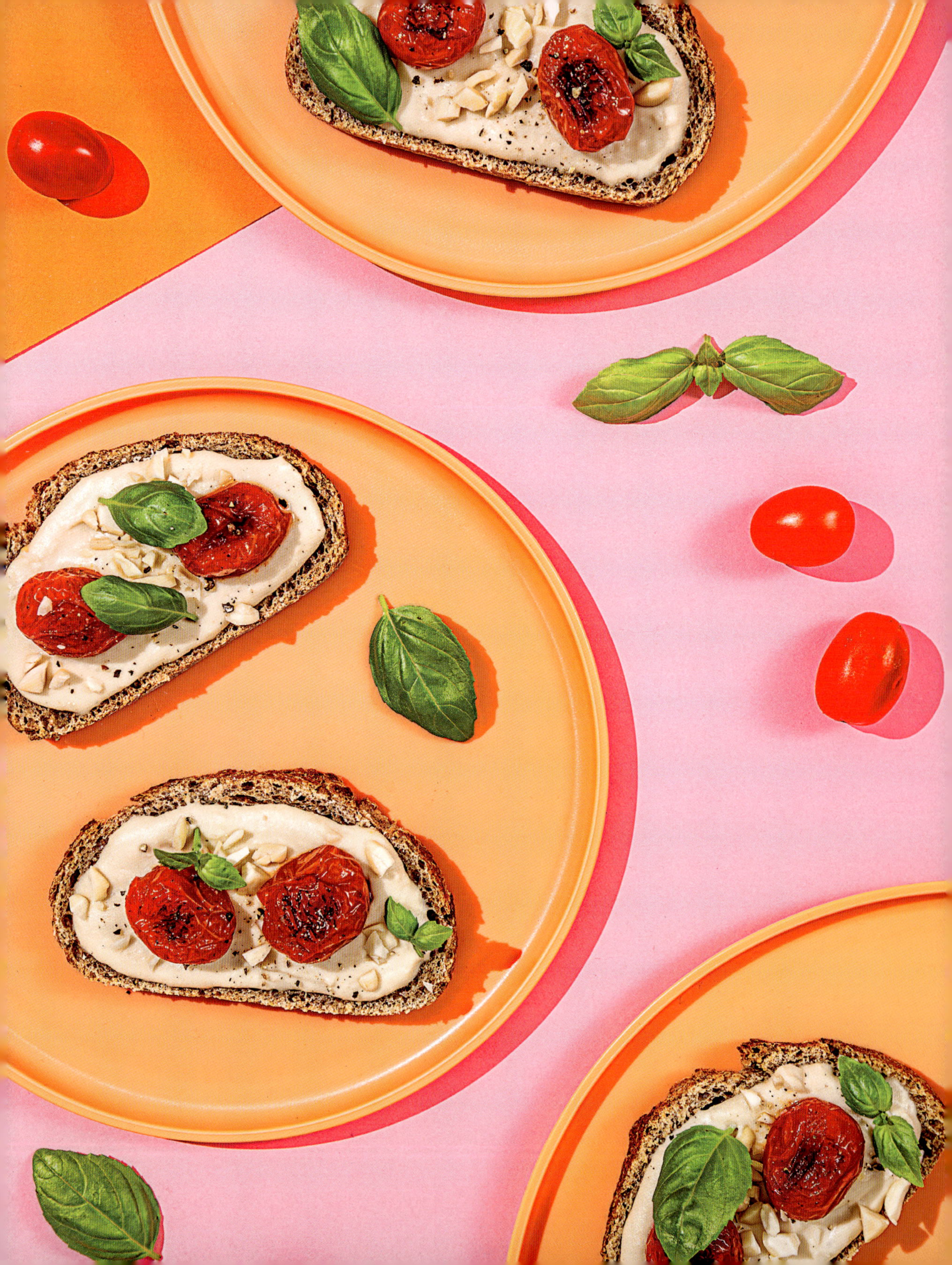

# BRUSCHETTA WITH WHITE BEAN AND ALMOND PASTE

- FOR 4 PEOPLE
- PREP/COOK TIME: 30 MIN
- SUMMER, OR ALL SEASONS WITHOUT CHERRY TOMATOES

**FOR THE PASTE**

3 tablespoons **olive oil**, divided
8 **cherry tomatoes**, cut in half
½ (15-ounce) can (200 grams) **white beans**, drained and rinsed
1 **clove garlic**, minced
**juice of ½ lemon**
1 tablespoon **almond butter**

**FOR THE TOPPING**

4 slices **whole wheat bread**
a few leaves **fresh basil**
2 tablespoons **almonds**, chopped
a drizzle of **olive oil**
**salt** and **pepper**, to taste

**1.** Preheat a skillet over medium heat with 1 tablespoon of olive oil. Add the cherry tomatoes to the pan and cook until slightly caramelized and starting to burst.

**2.** In a blender, combine the white beans, minced garlic, lemon juice, almond butter, salt, and pepper. Mix until creamy and consistent. Add the remaining olive oil, if necessary, to achieve the desired consistency.

**3.** Toast the slices of whole wheat bread.

**4.** Spread the white bean paste generously on the toasted bread slices.

**5.** Arrange the caramelized cherry tomatoes on top of the white bean paste.

**6.** Garnish with fresh basil leaves and chopped almonds.

**7.** Season with a drizzle of olive oil, salt, and pepper to taste.

FOR 100 G

| protein: **5.3 g** | carbohydrates: **20 g** | lipids: **5.4 g** |
|---|---|---|

PER SERVING (140 G)

| protein: **9.6 g** | carbohydrates: **35.9 g** | lipids: **9.8 g** |
|---|---|---|

# CASHEW LOLLIPOPS

FOR 4 PEOPLE (12 BALLS) · PREP/COOK TIME: 30 MIN · REST TIME: 20 MIN IN THE FREEZER · ALL SEASONS

**· 1⅓ cups (200 grams) cashews, whole · ¼ cup soy cooking cream · 3 tablespoons apple cider vinegar · juice of ¼ lemon · 2 teaspoons garlic powder · 1 teaspoon dried minced onions · 1 tablespoon herbes de provence · 2 cups (200 grams) mix of pistachios and walnuts, chopped · salt and pepper**

**1.** Start by soaking the cashews in hot water for at least 30 minutes. **2.** Then drain the cashews and transfer them to a blender, adding all other ingredients, except the mix of pistachios and nuts. **3.** Blend everything until you get a fairly smooth paste. **4.** Transfer the paste into a bowl and leave to rest in the freezer for about 20 minutes until slightly hardened. **5.** Meanwhile, roughly blend the pistachios and walnuts until chopped. **6.** Take the paste out of the freezer and form small balls in the palm of your hand. Then roll them in the chopped pistachios and walnuts to cover the plant-based "cheese." **7.** To serve, stick a small toothpick in each ball. Then let them sit in a cool place until ready to serve.

FOR 100 G

| protein: **16.7 g** | carbohydrates: **21.5 g** | lipids: **46.5 g** |
|---|---|---|

PER SERVING (130 G)

| protein: **21.7 g** | carbohydrates: **28 g** | lipids: **60.5 g** |
|---|---|---|

---

# PUMPKIN SEED AND CHICKPEA "SKYR"

FOR 2 PEOPLE · PREP/COOK TIME: 20 MIN · ALL SEASONS

**· 1¼ cups (150 grams) raw pumpkin seeds · 2 tablespoons lemon juice · 1 tablespoon apple cider vinegar · 1 tablespoon maple or agave syrup · ¼ (15½-ounce) can (100 grams) chickpeas, drained and rinsed · 1 tablespoon olive oil · ¼ teaspoon ground smoked paprika · 1 tablespoon pumpkin seeds, for garnish · a few leaves fresh cilantro · a few pomegranate seeds (optional) · ¼ teaspoon salt · ¼ teaspoon ground black pepper**

**1.** Soak the pumpkin seeds in water for at least 4 hours, ideally overnight. Then drain them and rinse them with clear water. **2.** Blend the pumpkin seeds with the lemon juice, apple cider vinegar, maple or agave syrup, salt, and black pepper until smooth and creamy. If necessary, add a little water to adjust the consistency. Set aside. **3.** Preheat the oven to 350°F. **4.** Drain and rinse the chickpeas. Dry them with a clean cloth. **5.** In a bowl, mix the chickpeas with the olive oil, ground smoked paprika, salt, and black pepper. **6.** Spread the seasoned chickpeas on a baking sheet covered with parchment paper and bake for 15 to 20 minutes. Stir them halfway through cooking. **7.** Spread the pumpkin seed "skyr" on plates and top with the cooled chickpeas. **8.** Sprinkle with pumpkin seeds, pomegranate seeds, if using, and fresh cilantro.

FOR 100 G

| protein: **14.1 g** | carbohydrates: **12.7 g** | lipids: **18.6 g** |
|---|---|---|

PER PORTION (170 G)

| protein: **24 g** | carbohydrates: **21.6 g** | lipids: **24.2 g** |
|---|---|---|

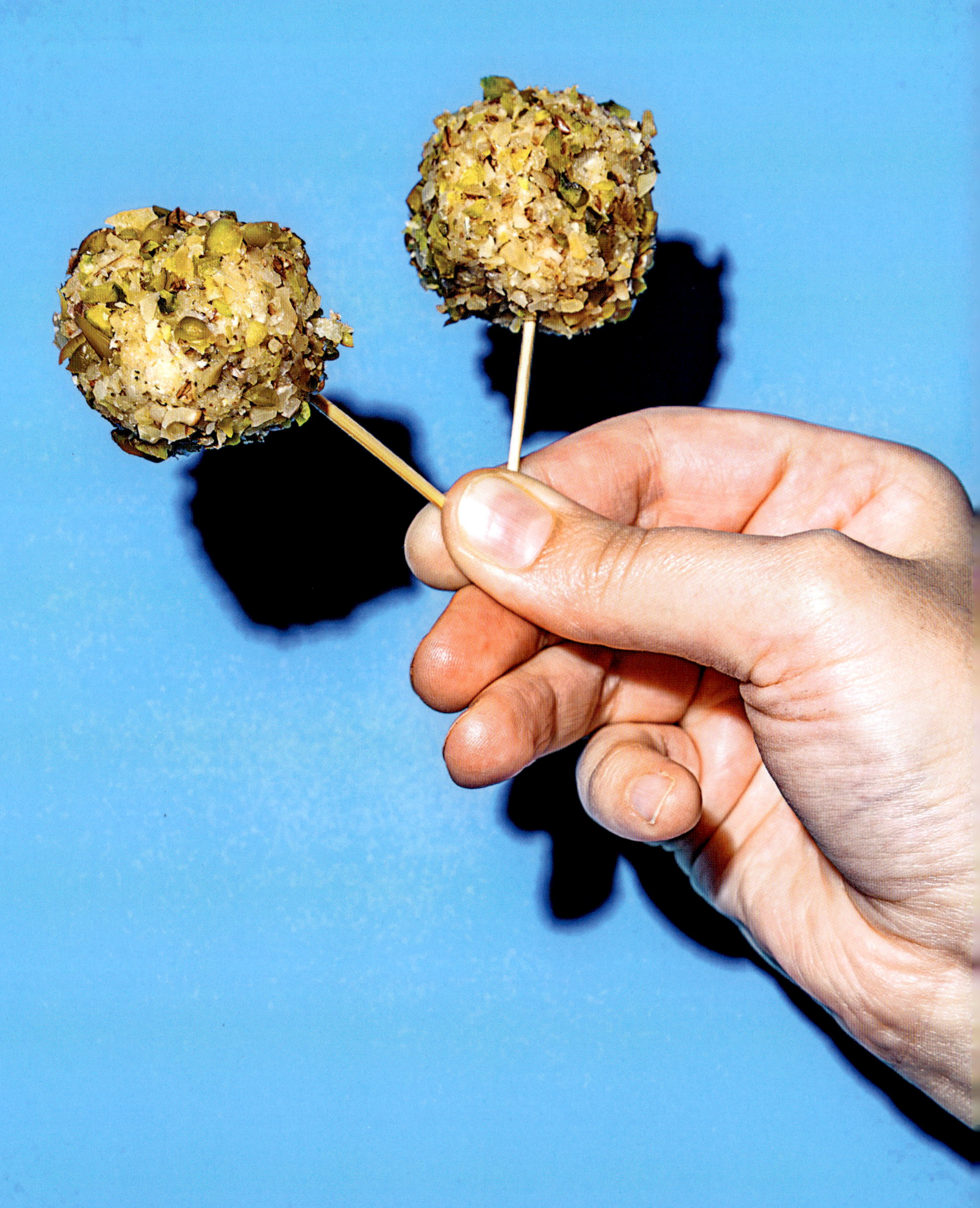

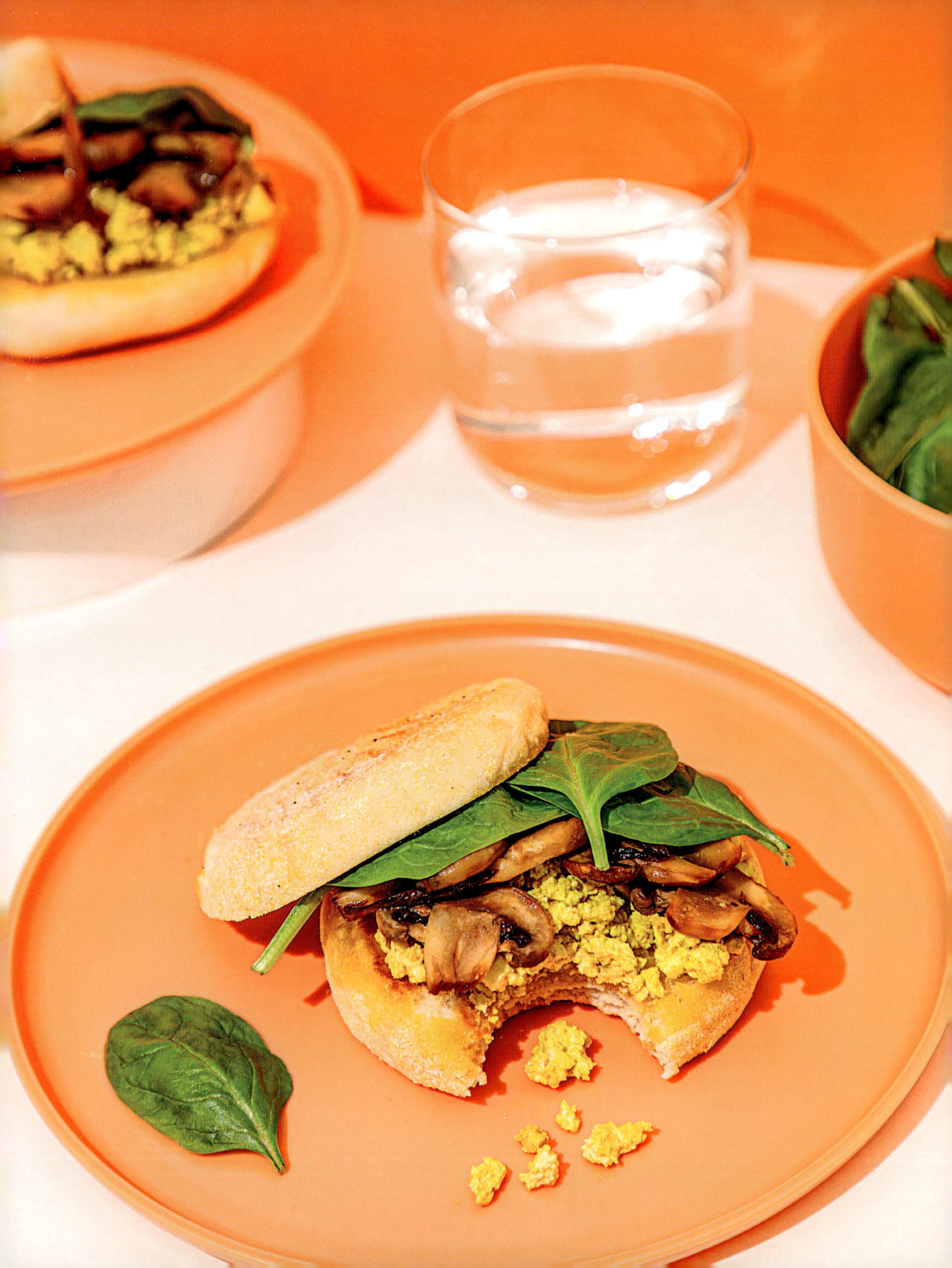

# ENGLISH MUFFIN WITH SCRAMBLED TOFU

- FOR 2 PEOPLE
- PREP/COOK TIME: 30 MIN
- ALL SEASONS

**FOR THE SCRAMBLED TOFU**
7 ounces (200 grams) **firm tofu**
2 tablespoons **olive oil**
3½ ounces (100 grams) **soft tofu**
2 teaspoons **ground turmeric**
**garlic powder**, to taste
1 tablespoon **soy sauce**

**FOR THE TOPPING**
1 large **onion**, chopped
1 teaspoon **sugar**
5 ounces (150 grams) **white mushrooms**
1 tablespoon **soy sauce**
3½ ounces (100 grams) **fresh spinach**

**TO SERVE**
2 **English muffins**

**1.** Press the firm tofu to remove the excess water and crumble it into a bowl, either with your fingers or a fork.

**2.** In a frying pan, heat 1 tablespoon of olive oil over low heat. Add the crumbled tofu and soft tofu and mix well to obtain a scrambled texture. Add the ground turmeric and garlic powder and mix well until the yellow color is evenly distributed. Then deglaze with 1 tablespoon of soy sauce, stirring until the tofu is well coated. Reserve and keep warm.

**3.** In the same pan, caramelize the chopped onion with 1 tablespoon of olive oil and sugar until golden and tender. Meanwhile, slice the mushrooms and add them to the pan. Cook for about 5 minutes and deglaze again with 1 tablespoon of soy sauce.

**4.** Wash and drain the fresh spinach and toast the English muffins in the toaster until golden and crispy.

**5.** On the bottom half of each English muffin, spread the scrambled tofu, sautéed mushrooms and onions, and fresh spinach. Cover everything with the other half of the English muffins. You can place them in the oven for a few minutes to reheat them if you wish or eat them immediately!

## Tips

- If you don't have soft tofu, you can use ½ cup of soy cooking cream instead.
- Adapt this recipe with other vegetables of your choice or add some plant-based "cheese" for an extra treat.

FOR 100 G

| protein: **8.5 g** | carbohydrates: **13.3 g** | lipids: **6.1 g** |
|---|---|---|

PER SERVING (380 G)

| protein: **32.8 g** | carbohydrates: **51.2 g** | lipids: **23.4 g** |
|---|---|---|

- **FOR 2 PEOPLE**
- **PREP/COOK TIME: 30 MIN**
- **ALL SEASONS**

# ENGLISH BREAKFAST

7 ounces (200 grams) **white mushrooms**
⅓ cup **olive oil**, divided
4 slices **plant-based "bacon"**
4 slices **whole wheat bread**
½ (15-ounce) can (200 grams) **baked beans**
1¼ cups (100 grams) **chickpea flour**
2 tablespoons **nutritional yeast**
**fresh spinach**
**salt** and **pepper**, divided

**1.** Preheat the oven to 400°F. On a baking sheet covered with baking paper, place your mushrooms cut into quarters and drizzle them with 1 tablespoon of olive oil. Sprinkle them with salt and pepper. Add the slices of plant-based "bacon" and whole wheat bread. Drizzle the bread with 2 tablespoons of olive oil.

**2.** Bake in the oven for 15 to 20 minutes until the mushrooms are tender, the bread is golden, and the "bacon" is crispy. Be careful: The mushrooms release juice, so keep them away from other foods!

**3.** Meanwhile, heat the baked beans in a saucepan over low heat.

**4.** Prepare your vegetable omelet by mixing the chickpea flour, nutritional yeast, and some salt and pepper in a bowl. Add water until smooth. Pour the batter into a hot oiled pan and cook until the vegetable omelet is firm on both sides.

**5.** Cook the spinach for a few minutes in a pan adding the remaining olive oil, salt, and pepper.

**6.** Place the beans, spinach, mushrooms, plant-based "bacon," veggie omelet, and toasted bread slices on plates in an artistic way!

FOR 100 G

| protein: **9.5 g** | carbohydrates: **23.7 g** | lipids: **5.2 g** |
|---|---|---|

PER PORTION (420 G)

| protein: **40.1 g** | carbohydrates: **94.9 g** | lipids: **21.9 g** |
|---|---|---|

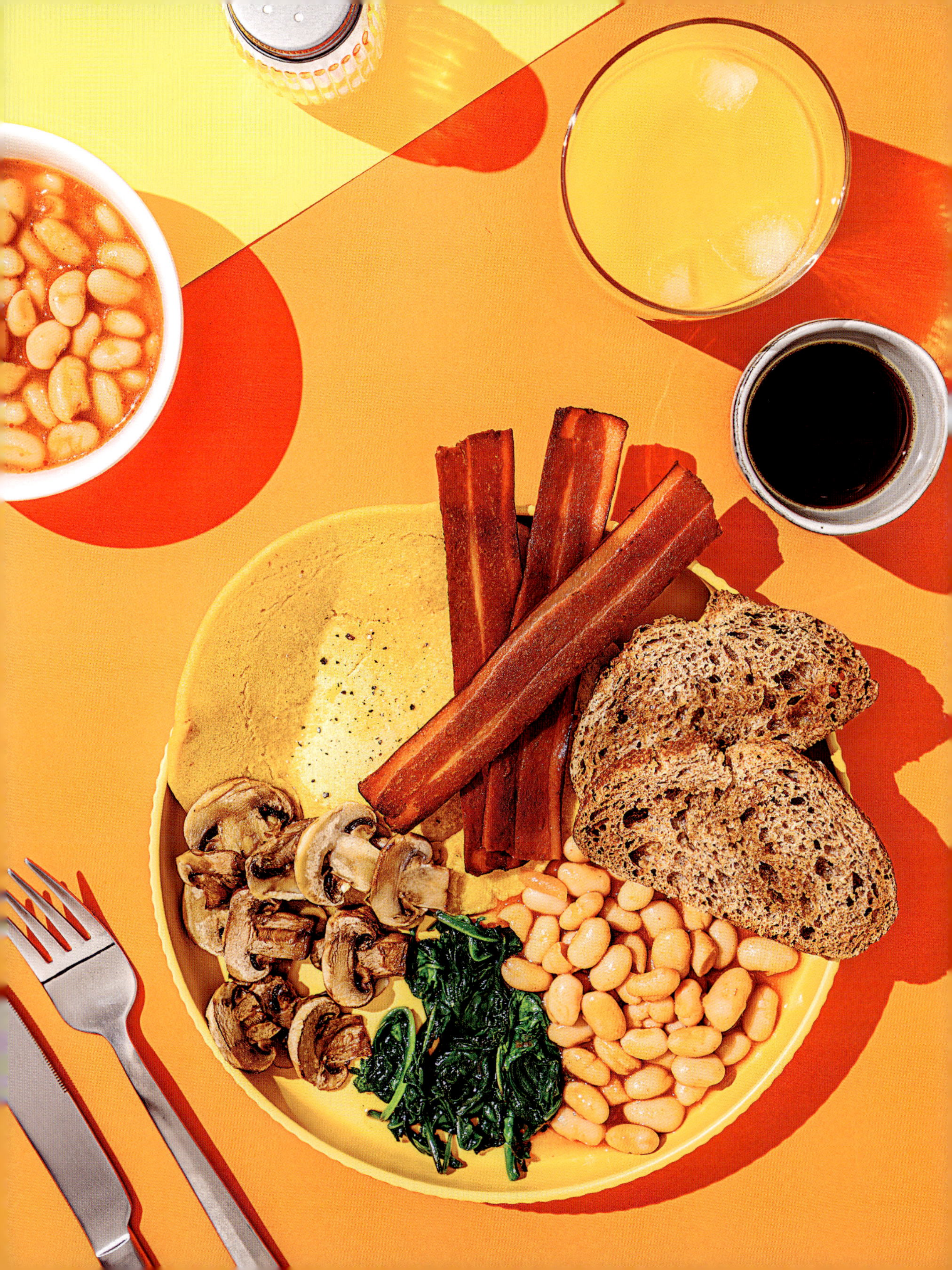

- FOR 2 PEOPLE
- PREP/COOK TIME: 30 MIN
- ALL SEASONS

# PLANT-BASED CROQUE MONSIEUR

**FOR THE BÉCHAMEL**

2 tablespoons (30 grams) **plant butter**, unsalted
2 tablespoons **olive oil**
¼ cup (30 grams) all-purpose **flour**
1 cup (250 milliliters) **soy milk**
**salt** and **pepper**
a pinch of **nutmeg**
2 tablespoons **nutritional yeast**

**FOR THE TOAST**

4 large slices **whole wheat bread**
2 tablespoons **plant butter**, unsalted
2 slices **plant-based "ham"**
½ cup (50 grams) **plant-based grated "cheese"**

**TO SERVE**

**green salad**

**1.** Preheat the oven to 350°F.

**2.** To prepare the béchamel, melt the plant butter in a saucepan over medium heat and add the olive oil. Add the flour and stir well for about 1 minute to make a roux. Then add the soy milk a little bit at a time, stirring constantly until the sauce thickens. Season with salt, pepper, and nutmeg and add the nutritional yeast. Then remove from the heat and set aside.

**3.** On 2 slices of whole wheat bread, spread plant butter, place a slice of plant-based "ham," and sprinkle with ⅔ of the plant-based grated "cheese." Top with the remaining 2 slices of bread to form 2 sandwiches.

**4.** On top of the sandwiches, generously pour béchamel sauce, then sprinkle with the rest of the plant-based grated "cheese."

**5.** Place the plant-based croque monsieurs on a baking sheet and bake for about 10 to 15 minutes, until golden and crispy.

**6.** Once cooked, remove the plant-based croque monsieurs from the oven and cut them in half. Arrange them on plates and serve with green salad.

## Tip

You can also cut thin slices of smoked tofu and pan fry them with ground paprika and garlic powder to replace the plant-based "ham."

FOR 100 G

| protein: **9.9 g** | carbohydrates: **26 g** | lipids: **19.8 g** |
|---|---|---|

PER PORTION (240 G)

| protein: **23.9 g** | carbohydrates: **62.9 g** | lipids: **47.9 g** |
|---|---|---|

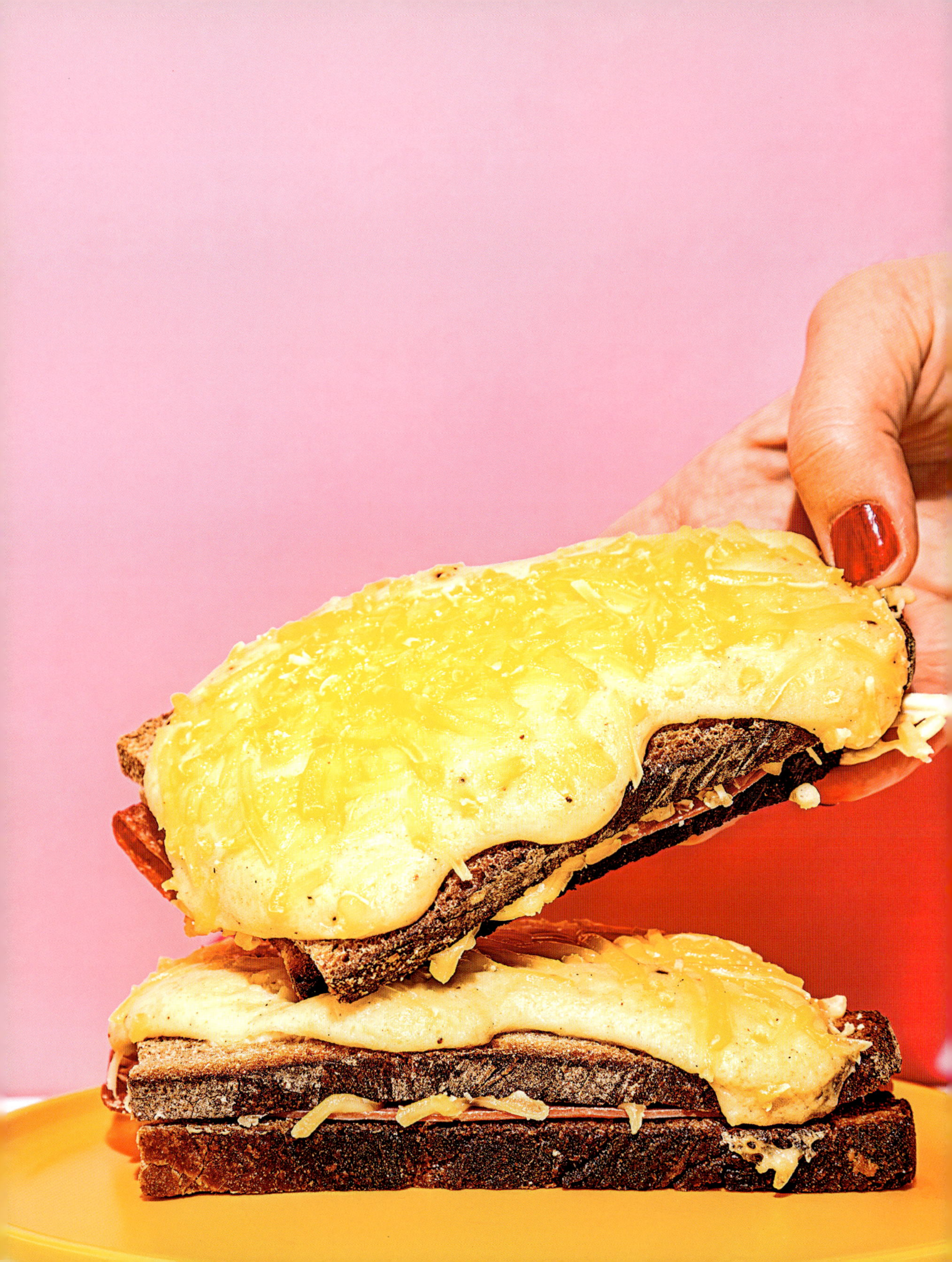

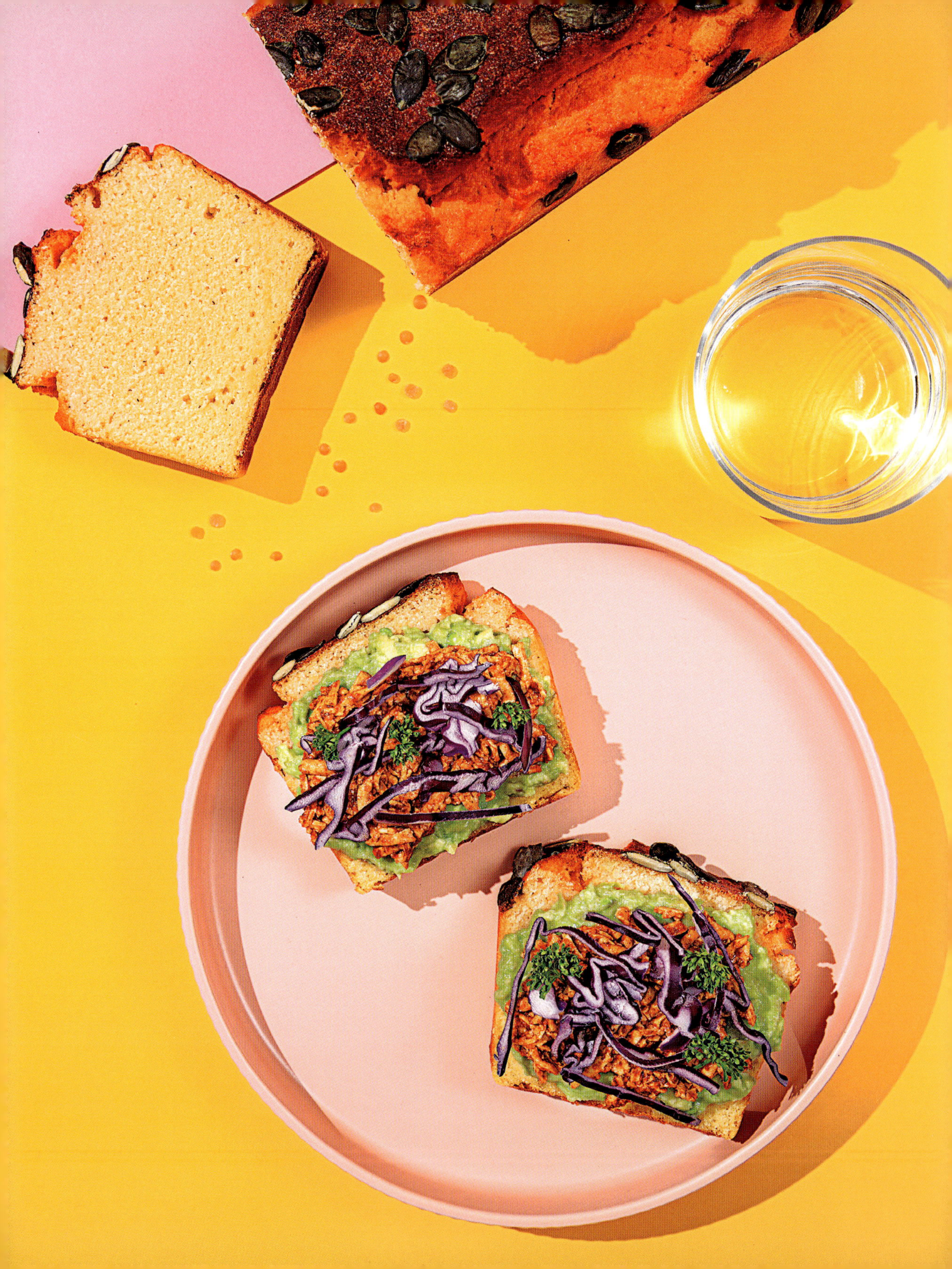

# LENTIL, AVOCADO, AND TOFU BREAD

- FOR 2 PEOPLE
- PREP/COOK TIME: 1 HOUR
- REST TIME: 1 NIGHT
- ALL SEASONS

**FOR THE RED LENTIL BREAD**
2½ cups (500 grams) **red lentils**
3/4 cup **water**
1 (¼-ounce) bag **active dry yeast**
¼ cup (50 grams) **olive oil**
1 teaspoon **fine salt**
a handful of **pumpkin seeds**

**FOR THE GRATED TOFU**
6 ounces (180 grams) **firm tofu**
2 teaspoons **ground smoked paprika**
1 teaspoon **garlic powder**
1 tablespoon **olive oil**
2 tablespoons **barbecue sauce**

**TO SERVE**
1 **avocado**, mashed
¼ **red cabbage**, thinly sliced
a few leaves **fresh parsley**, chopped
**salt** and **pepper**

**1.** Soak the lentils overnight. Then drain them and rinse them before transferring them to a blender with ¾ cup of water, the yeast, the oil, and the salt. Blend until you get a smooth paste.

**2.** In a deep cake pan, place some baking paper, then pour in the lentil bread paste. Sprinkle pumpkin seeds evenly on top. Let sit in a warm, dry place for 30 to 40 minutes to allow the yeast to work. Then bake your lentil bread paste in the oven at 350°F for 40 to 50 minutes. Monitor regularly during cooking: Your lentil bread is ready when a toothpick comes out clean after inserting it in the middle.

**3.** While the lentil bread is baking, grate the tofu. Then place it in a bowl and add the ground smoked paprika, garlic powder, olive oil, and barbecue sauce. Mix well before spreading it on a baking sheet covered with baking paper. Bake in the oven for about 20 minutes, stirring halfway through cooking. If it becomes too dry, add a little more barbecue sauce.

**4.** When the lentil bread and tofu are ready, cut 2 nice slices of bread and spread with the previously mashed avocado. Top each slice with the tofu and thinly sliced red cabbage. Sprinkle with fresh parsley and adjust the seasoning with salt and pepper to taste.

## Tips

- Be careful—some commercial barbecue sauces contain anchovies... Check carefully that your barbecue sauce is plant based.
- Once this high-protein bread is made, store it in a dry place.

FOR 100 G

| protein: **6.2 g** | carbohydrates: **9.8 g** | lipids: **9.5 g** |
|---|---|---|

PER SERVING (370 G)

| protein: **23 g** | carbohydrates: **36.4 g** | lipids: **35.3 g** |
|---|---|---|

# VEGETABLE SPREAD

**FOR 4 PEOPLE • PREP/COOK TIME: 10 MIN • ALL SEASONS**

**• 1 (15½-ounce) can (400 grams) chickpeas, drained and rinsed • 4 artichoke hearts, drained • juice of ½ lemon • 2 tablespoons avocado mayonnaise • 1 tablespoon tamari • 2 teaspoons tomato paste • 1 tablespoon olive oil • salt and pepper, to taste**

**1.** In a blender, place the drained and rinsed chickpeas. **2.** Add the drained artichoke hearts, lemon juice, avocado mayonnaise, tamari, tomato paste, and olive oil. **3.** Roughly blend all ingredients to maintain a uniform texture. **4.** Keep cool before serving on whole wheat toast.

**Tip:** You can also enjoy this vegetable spread as a dip by dipping in raw vegetable sticks.

FOR 100 G

| protein: **5.3 g** | carbohydrates: **16.8 g** | lipids: **6.6 g** |
|---|---|---|

PER PORTION (180 G)

| protein: **9.4 g** | carbohydrates: **29.8 g** | lipids: **11.7 g** |
|---|---|---|

---

# LENTIL AND WALNUT TERRINE

**FOR 4 PEOPLE • PREP/COOK TIME: 25 MIN • ALL SEASONS**

**• 2 tablespoons olive oil, divided • 1 onion, finely chopped • 2 cloves garlic, minced • 2¾ cups (200 grams) lentils, cooked • ¾ cup (100 grams) walnuts, chopped • 1 teaspoon mustard • 2 tablespoons soy sauce • 2 tablespoons nutritional yeast • slices of whole wheat bread • pickles • salt and ground black pepper, to taste**

**1.** Heat 1 tablespoon of olive oil in a skillet over medium heat. Add the onion and sauté for about 5 minutes, until golden and lightly caramelized. **2.** Add the minced garlic to the pan and sauté for an additional 1 to 2 minutes, until the garlic is lightly browned and fragrant. Remove the pan from the heat and let cool slightly. **3.** In a blender, combine cooked lentils, walnuts, sautéed onion, garlic, mustard, soy sauce, remaining olive oil, and nutritional yeast. Season with salt and ground black pepper to taste. Roughly mix all ingredients. **4.** Place the mixture in an airtight container and let cool in the fridge for at least 1 hour. **5.** Once the terrine has cooled, you can serve it on slices of whole wheat bread with pickles.

FOR 100 G

| protein: **9.6 g** | carbohydrates: **15.4 g** | lipids: **19.4 g** |
|---|---|---|

PER PORTION (120 G)

| protein: **11.7 g** | carbohydrates: **18.7 g** | lipids: **23.6 g** |
|---|---|---|

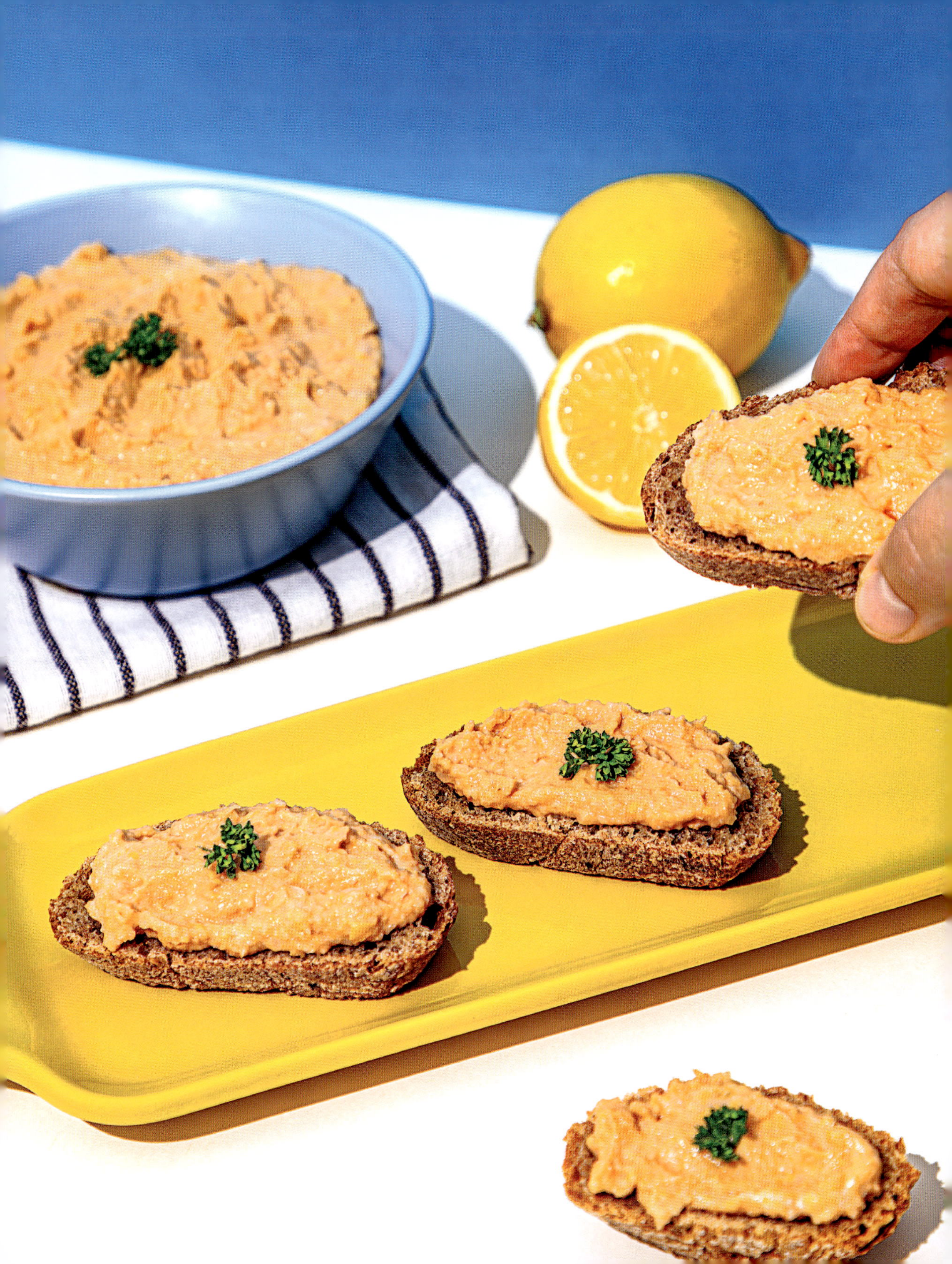

# SWEET SNACKS

- FOR 6 PEOPLE
- PREP/COOK TIME: 35 MIN
- ALL SEASONS

# CHICKPEA AND PEANUT BUTTER BROWNIES

1 teaspoon **plant butter**, unsalted (optional)
½ (15½-ounce) can (200 grams) **chickpeas**, drained and rinsed
⅓ cup (40 grams) **whole wheat flour**
2 tablespoons **vegan chocolate protein powder** (optional)
1 tablespoon **cocoa powder**
2 tablespoons **peanut butter**
½ cup (15 centiliters) **milk alternative** (soy, oat, . . .)
2¾ tablespoons **sugar**
1 teaspoon **vanilla extract**
1 tablespoon **baking powder**
½ tablespoon **coconut flakes**

**1.** Preheat the oven to 400°F. Lightly grease a brownie pan with plant butter or line it with baking paper to prevent sticking.

**2.** In a blender, combine the drained chickpeas, whole wheat flour, chocolate protein powder, cocoa powder, peanut butter, milk alternative, sugar, vanilla extract, and baking powder. Blend until you obtain a smooth batter without lumps.

**3.** Pour the batter into the prepared pan, making sure to smooth the surface with a spatula. Sprinkle the coconut flakes evenly over the surface of the batter.

**4.** Place the pan in the center of the preheated oven and bake the brownies for about 20 minutes or until cooked through. To check the brownies are cooked, insert a toothpick into the middle—it should come out clean.

**5.** Once cooked, remove the brownies from the oven and let cool in the pan for a few minutes.

**6.** Carefully remove the brownies using the baking paper or a spatula, then leave to cool for 15 minutes. Once cooled, cut into squares, and ready!

## Tip

You can adjust the recipe by using different milk alternatives to change the flavor. You can also use kidney beans instead of chickpeas.

FOR 100 G

| protein: **9.7 g** (or **6.7g** without protein powder) | carbohydrates: **26.5 g** | lipids: **5.6 g** |
|---|---|---|

PER SERVING (85 G)

| protein: **8.2 g** (or **5.7g** without protein powder) | carbohydrates: **22.5 g** | lipids: **4.8 g** |
|---|---|---|

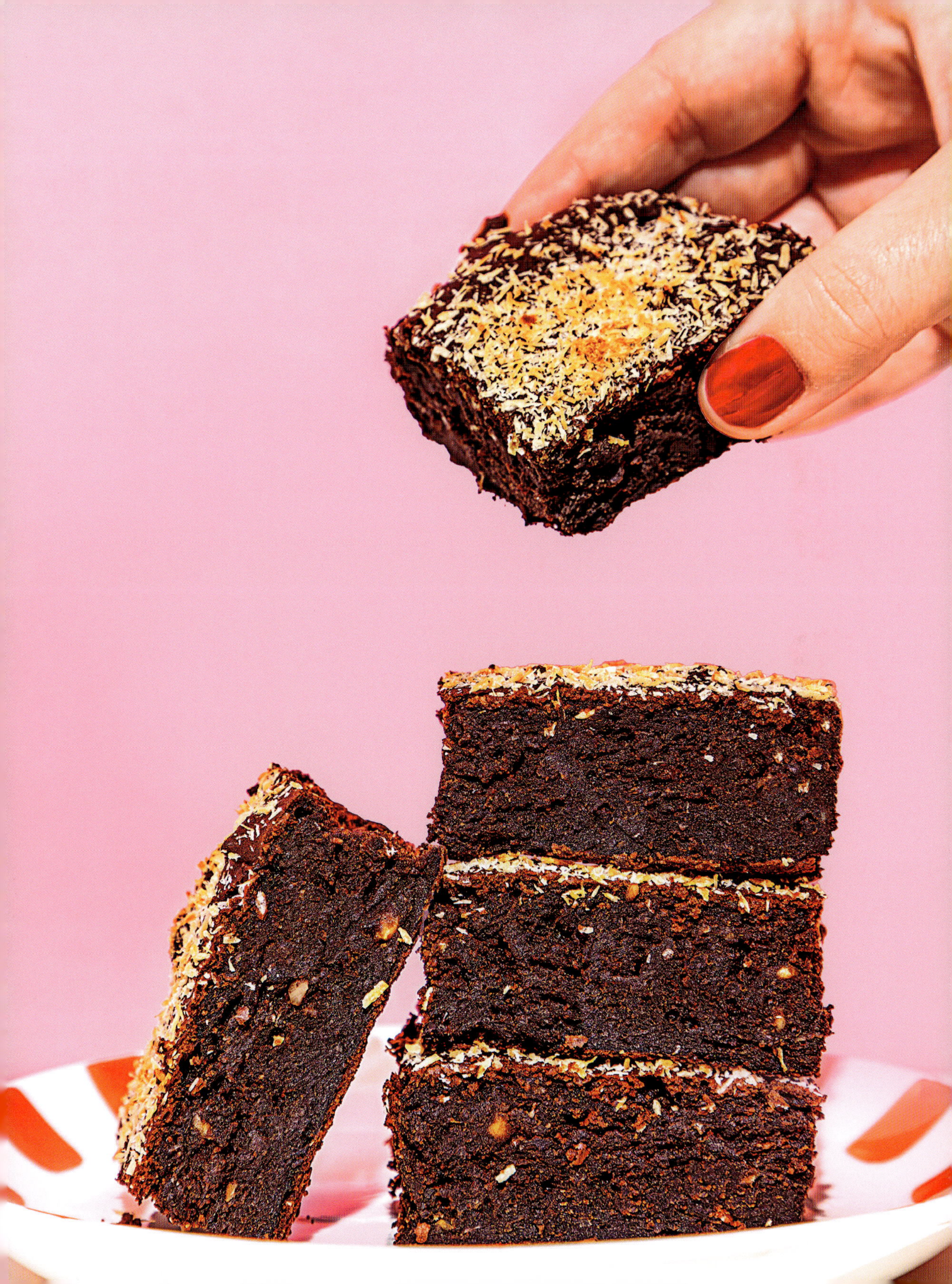

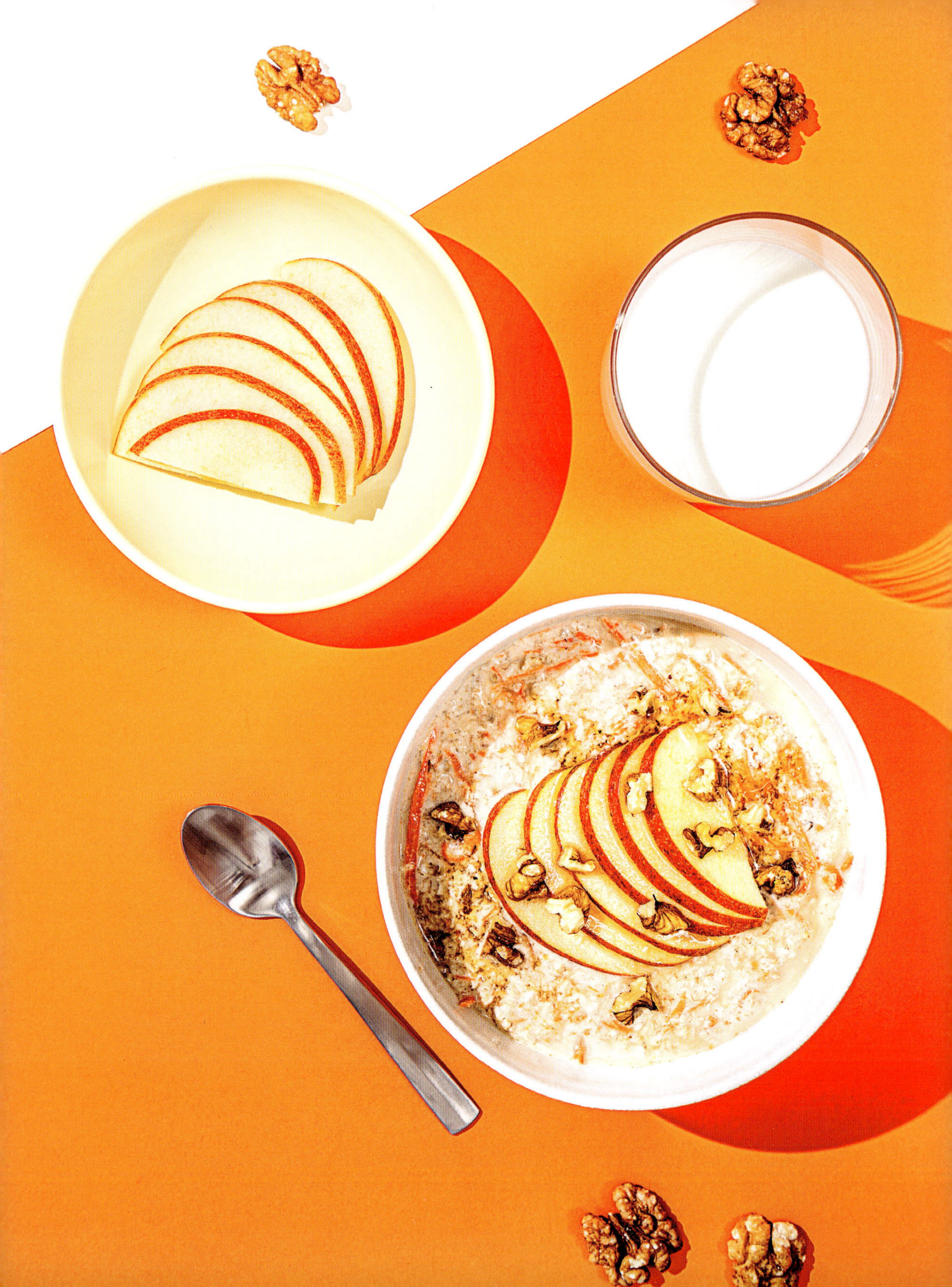

# CARROT CAKE OATMEAL

**FOR 2 PEOPLE • PREP/COOK TIME: 10 MIN • REST TIME: 4 HOURS TO 1 NIGHT IN THE FRIDGE • ALL SEASONS**

**• 1 medium carrot, grated • 1 cup (90 grams) oats • 1 tablespoon raisins and chopped nuts • 1 cup (240 milliliters) soy milk • 2 tablespoons maple syrup • ½ teaspoon ground cinnamon • ¼ teaspoon ground ginger • a pinch of nutmeg • a pinch of salt**

**1.** In a bowl, mix all ingredients. Stir well. **2.** Cover the bowl and place it in the refrigerator overnight, or for at least 4 hours, to allow time for the flavors to develop and the oats to soften. **3.** The next morning, remove the oatmeal from the refrigerator and stir. If the oatmeal is too thick, you can add a little more soy milk to reach the desired consistency. **4.** Reheat the oatmeal in the microwave or in a saucepan if you prefer to eat it hot, or enjoy it as is.

**Tip:** When serving, you can add additional toppings such as fresh fruit or an extra drizzle of maple syrup.

FOR 100 G

| protein: **4.5 g** | carbohydrates: **23.7 g** | lipids: **3.0 g** |
|---|---|---|

PER PORTION (220 G)

| protein: **10.1 g** | carbohydrates: **53.2 g** | lipids: **6.7 g** |
|---|---|---|

---

# CHIA PUDDING

**FOR 1 PERSON • PREP/COOK TIME: 10 MIN • REST TIME: 20 MIN TO 1 NIGHT IN THE FRIDGE • ALL SEASONS**

**• 2 tablespoons chia seeds • ¾ cup (20 centiliters) soy milk • mix of nuts (almonds, cashews, walnuts, etc.) • seasonal fruits**

**1.** Pour the chia seeds and the soy into a large glass or bowl. Stir the mixture well for the first 10 minutes to prevent the chia seeds from clumping together. **2.** As soon as the chia seeds start to absorb the liquid, place them in the refrigerator. Let rest for at least 20 minutes, ideally overnight for an optimal texture. **3.** Meanwhile, prepare your toppings by choosing a combination of fresh fruit and dried fruit. For example, slice some strawberries and chop some cashew nuts. **4.** Remove the chia pudding from the refrigerator and gently mix in the toppings or arrange them nicely on top, depending on your preference.

**Tip:** Depending on your taste, you can use a sweetener, like jam or agave syrup.

FOR 100 G

| protein: **6.3 g** | carbohydrates: **8.6 g** | lipids: **11.7 g** |
|---|---|---|

PER SERVING (260 G)

| protein: **16.3 g** | carbohydrates: **22.2 g** | lipids: **30.3 g** |
|---|---|---|

- FOR 4 PEOPLE
- PREP TIME: 30 MIN
- ALL SEASONS

# SPELT AND BANANA PANCAKES

**FOR THE PANCAKES**
1 cup (120 grams) **spelt flour**
2 tablespoons (30 grams) **vegan vanilla protein powder**
1 teaspoon **baking powder**
1 ripe **banana**
1 cup (240 milliliters) **almond milk**
1 tablespoon **melted coconut oil**
1 tablespoon **agave syrup**
a pinch of **salt**

**FOR THE TOPPING**
**seasonal fruits**
**agave** or **maple syrup**

**1.** In a large bowl, mix flour, protein powder, baking powder, and a pinch of salt.

**2.** In another bowl, mash the ripe banana until smooth. Add the almond milk and melted coconut oil. Then mix well.

**3.** Pour the liquid mixture into the bowl of dry ingredients and mix until well combined. If the batter is too thick, you can add a little more almond milk to reach the desired consistency.

**4.** Heat a non-stick skillet over medium heat and pour a small ladle of batter to form a pancake. Let cook for about 2 to 3 minutes on each side, or until bubbles begin to form on the surface and the edges are lightly browned.

**5.** Repeat with the remaining batter until all the pancakes are ready.

**6.** Now you can coat them with agave or maple syrup and garnish them with the toppings of your choice.

FOR 100 G

| protein: **7.4 g** | carbohydrates: **25.1 g** | lipids: **4.7 g** |
|---|---|---|

PER SERVING (140 G)

| protein: **10.2 g** | carbohydrates: **34.5 g** | lipids: **6.5 g** |
|---|---|---|

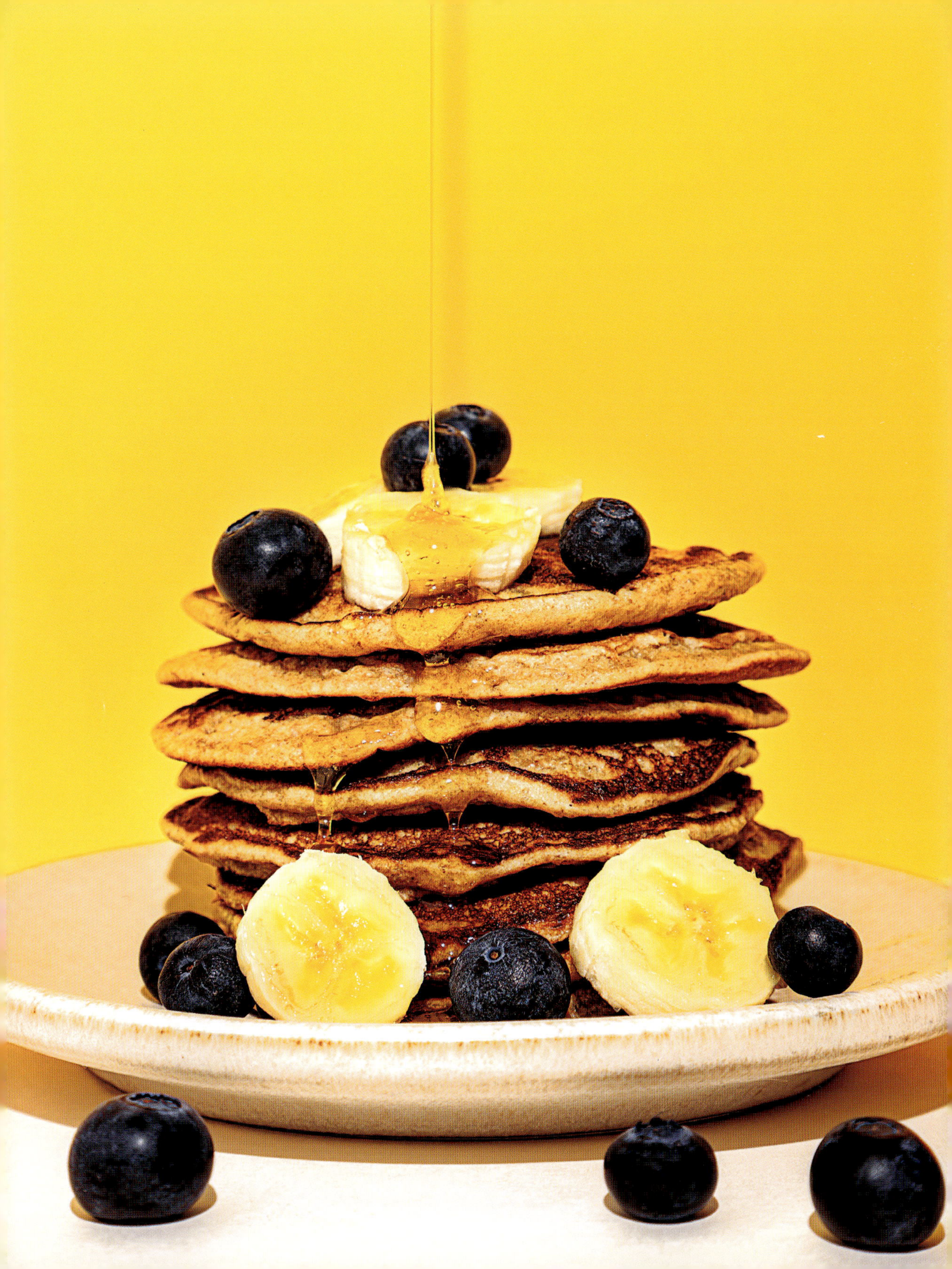

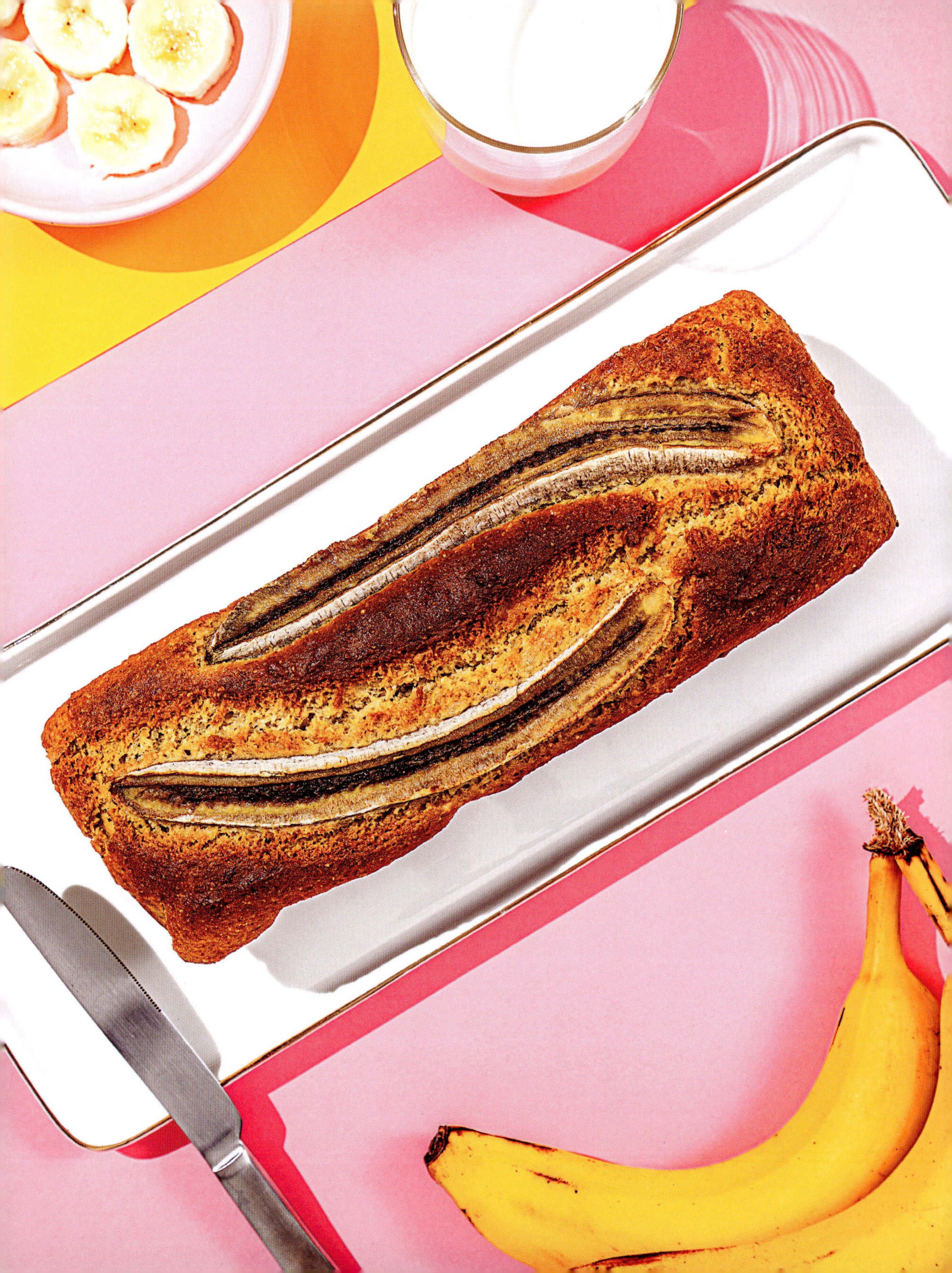

# BANANA BREAD WITH ALMOND CUSTARD

- FOR 6 PEOPLE
- PREP/COOK TIME: 1 HOUR
- ALL SEASONS

1 teaspoon **plant butter**, unsalted
2 or 3 ripe **bananas**, mashed
¼ cup (60 milliliters) **melted coconut oil** or **vegetable oil**
½ cup (100 grams) **cane sugar**
1 tablespoon **apple cider vinegar**
¼ cup (60 milliliters) **soy milk**
1 teaspoon **vanilla extract**
1½ cups (200 grams) **whole wheat flour**
1¼ cups (100 grams) **chickpea flour**
1 cup (100 grams) **almond flour**
1 teaspoon **baking soda**
1 teaspoon **baking powder**
1 teaspoon **ground cinnamon**
a pinch of **salt**

**1.** Preheat the oven to 350°F and lightly grease a cake pan with plant butter.

**2.** In a large bowl, mix mashed bananas, melted coconut oil, sugar, apple cider vinegar, soy milk, and vanilla extract.

**3.** In another bowl, mix the flours, baking soda, baking powder, ground cinnamon, and salt.

**4.** Gradually incorporate the dry ingredients into the banana mixture until the batter is smooth.

**5.** Pour the batter into the prepared cake pan and spread it evenly.

**6.** Bake the banana bread for 45 to 55 minutes, or until a toothpick inserted in the middle comes out clean.

**7.** Let the banana bread cool in the pan for about 10 minutes, then remove it from the pan, and let it cool before slicing and enjoying.

FOR 100 G

| protein: **8.6 g** | carbohydrates: **44.8 g** | lipids: **13.8 g** |
|---|---|---|

PER PORTION (170 G)

| protein: **14.6 g** | carbohydrates: **76.2 g** | lipids: **23.5 g** |
|---|---|---|

- FOR 2 PEOPLE
- PREP TIME: 10 MIN
- REST TIME: 30 MIN AT ROOM TEMPERATURE, 2 HOURS IN THE FRIDGE
- ALL SEASONS

# COCONUT-VANILLA PANNA COTTA

**FOR THE PANNA COTTA**

1 cup (200 milliliters) **coconut milk**
3⅓ tablespoons (40 grams) **coconut sugar** or **maple syrup**
1 teaspoon **vanilla extract**
7 ounces (200 grams) **soft tofu**
1 teaspoon **agar-agar**

**TO SERVE**

**fresh fruit** or **fruit coulis**

**1.** In a saucepan, mix the coconut milk, coconut sugar or maple syrup, and vanilla extract. Heat over medium heat until mixture is hot but not boiling, stirring to dissolve sugar or maple syrup.

**2.** At the same time, with an immersion blender, blend the soft tofu until you obtain a smooth and creamy texture (you can also loosen it with a whisk). Add the soft tofu to the pan and blend or whisk again, until well combined. Sprinkle the agar-agar on top and mix well to incorporate.

**3.** Bring the mixture to a boil, then reduce the heat and simmer for about 2 minutes, stirring constantly to prevent the mixture from sticking to the bottom of the pan.

**4.** Pour the mixture into ramekins and leave to cool at room temperature for about 30 minutes. Then place the ramekins in the refrigerator for at least 2 hours, or until the panna cotta is set.

**5.** Once ready, carefully transfer the panna cottas from the ramekins onto individual plates by placing the ramekins upside down on a plate. Serve the panna cottas with fresh fruit or a fruit coulis, if you wish.

## Tip

Let's compare like with like: Even if 4 grams of protein per 100 grams doesn't seem like a lot, it is necessary to remember that this is only a snack or dessert. Take a look at yogurts labeled "high in protein" in any grocery store: They show the exact same amount.

FOR 100 G

| protein: **4 g** | carbohydrates: **8.7 g** | lipids: **9 g** |
|---|---|---|

PER PORTION (220 G)

| protein: **8.8 g** | carbohydrates: **19.1 g** | lipids: **19.8 g** |
|---|---|---|

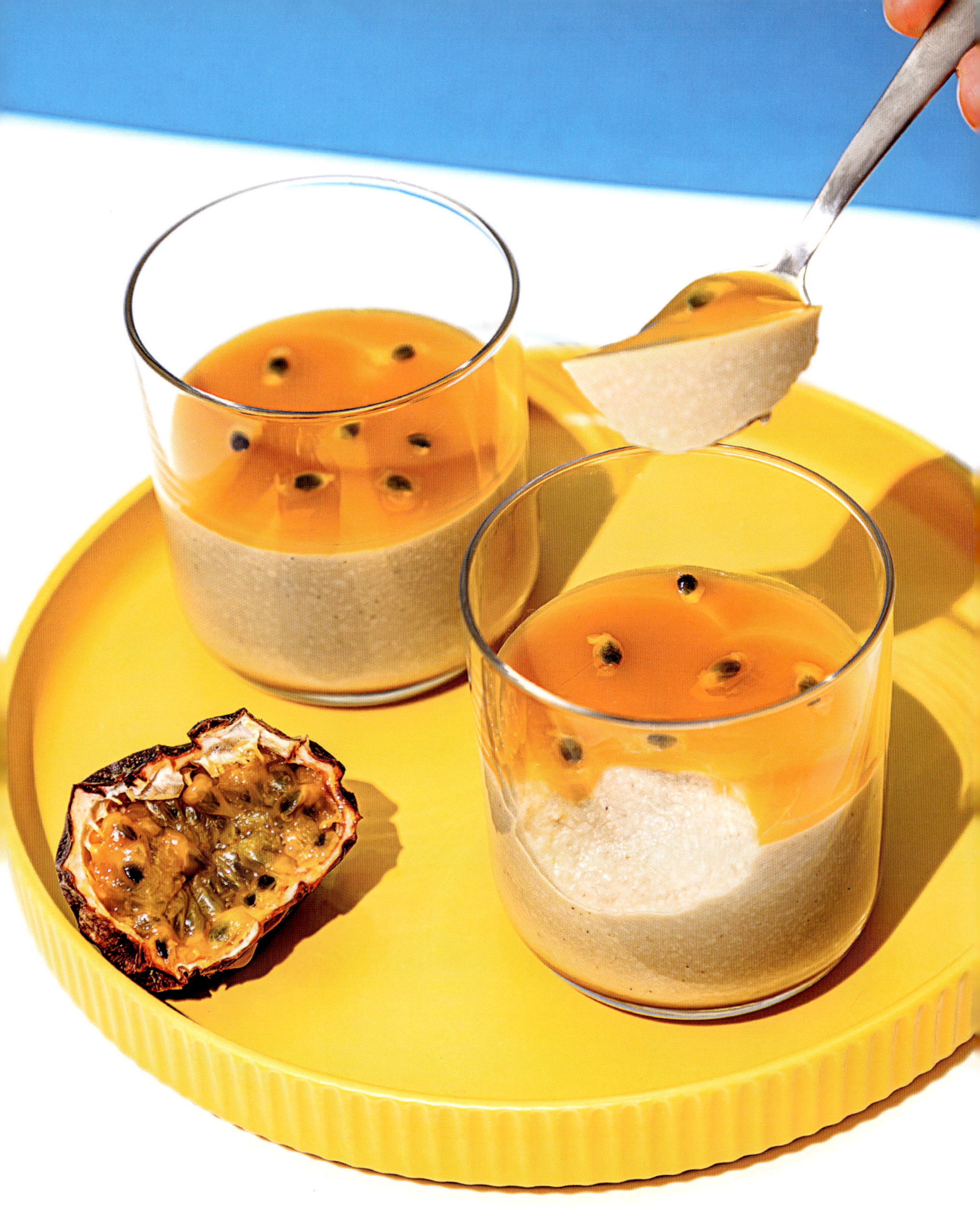

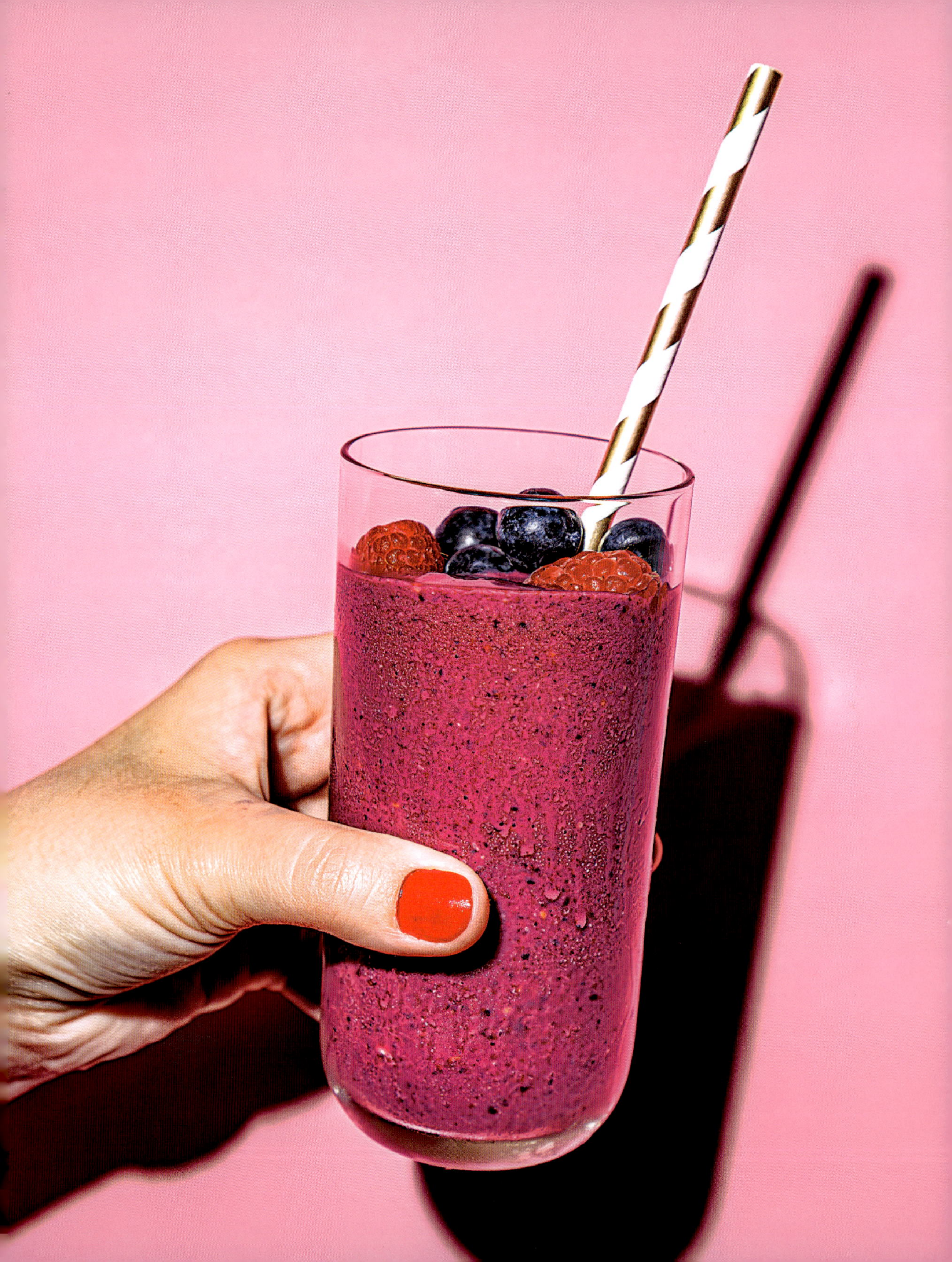

# RED SMOOTHIE WITH CHIA SEEDS

**FOR 2 PEOPLE • PREP/COOK TIME: 10 MIN • ALL SEASONS**

**• 1 ripe banana • 2 tablespoons almond butter • 1 cup (250 milliliters) soy milk • 1 cup (150 grams) frozen red berries (strawberries, raspberries, blackberries, blueberries) • 1 tablespoon vanilla protein powder • 1 tablespoon chia seeds**

**1.** Peel the banana and cut it into pieces. **2.** In a blender, add all ingredients. **3.** Blend all ingredients until you get a smooth and creamy texture. If the smoothie is too thick, you can add a little more soy milk to reach the desired consistency. **4.** You can add sweetener if you wish, but your smoothie is ready to drink.

| FOR 100 G | | |
|---|---|---|
| protein: **5.2 g** | carbohydrates: **10.7 g** | lipids: **5.5 g** |

| PER SERVING (290 G) | | |
|---|---|---|
| protein: **15.1 g** | carbohydrates: **31.1 g** | lipids: **16 g** |

---

# GREEN SMOOTHIE WITH SPINACH AND SPIRULINA

**FOR 2 PEOPLE • PREP/COOK TIME: 10 MIN • SUMMER**

**• 2 handfuls fresh spinach • ½ cucumber • ½ avocado • 1 ripe banana • 2 teaspoons spirulina powder • 2 tablespoons flax seeds • 1 cup (250 milliliters) soy milk • juice of ½ lemon • a few leaves fresh mint (optional) • a few ice cubes (optional)**

**1.** Start by carefully washing your fresh spinach. Then peel and roughly chop the cucumber, avocado, and banana. **2.** In a blender, add the spinach, spirulina, banana, avocado, flax seeds, and soy milk. **3.** Pour the lemon juice into the mixture. **4.** If you like, add a few mint leaves for a touch of freshness. **5.** Blend all ingredients until smooth and creamy. **6.** If you prefer, add a few ice cubes to make your smoothie cool and refreshing. You can also adjust the consistency with a little water or more soy milk.

| FOR 100 G | | |
|---|---|---|
| protein: **3.8 g** | carbohydrates: **7.8 g** | lipids: **4.9 g** |

| PER SERVING (290 G) | | |
|---|---|---|
| protein: **11.1 g** | carbohydrates: **22.8 g** | lipids: **14.3 g** |

- FOR 4 PEOPLE (8 CREPES)
- PREP/COOK TIME: 30 MIN
- REST TIME: 10 MIN
- ALL SEASONS

# THREE-INGREDIENT CREPE

**FOR THE CREPES**

2½ cups (300 grams) **all-purpose flour**
10½ ounces (300 grams) **soft tofu**
2½ cups (600 milliliters) **soy milk**

**FOR THE TOPPING**

seasonal **fresh fruits**
**maple syrup**

**1.** In a large bowl, pour the flour and then add the soft tofu.

**2.** Slowly pour the soy milk into the bowl, stirring constantly, until the batter is smooth and uniform. You can use a whisk to make mixing easier.

**3.** Let the batter rest for about 10 minutes to thicken slightly.

**4.** Meanwhile, heat a non-stick skillet over medium heat.

**5.** Once the skillet is hot, pour a ladleful of batter into it and tilt the skillet to distribute the batter evenly. Let the crepe cook for about 2 minutes, until bubbles begin to form on the surface. Flip the crepe and let the other side cook for 1 to 2 minutes, until lightly browned.

**6.** Repeat the process with the remaining batter.

**7.** Once all the crepes are cooked, serve them hot with fresh fruit and maple syrup, or your favorite toppings.

## Tip

The taste is neutral so you can eat them salty or sweet.

FOR 100 G

| protein: **5.8 g** | carbohydrates: **19.4 g** | lipids: **1.9 g** |
|---|---|---|

PER PORTION (300 G)

| protein: **17.4 g** | carbohydrates: **58.2 g** | lipids: **5.7 g** |
|---|---|---|

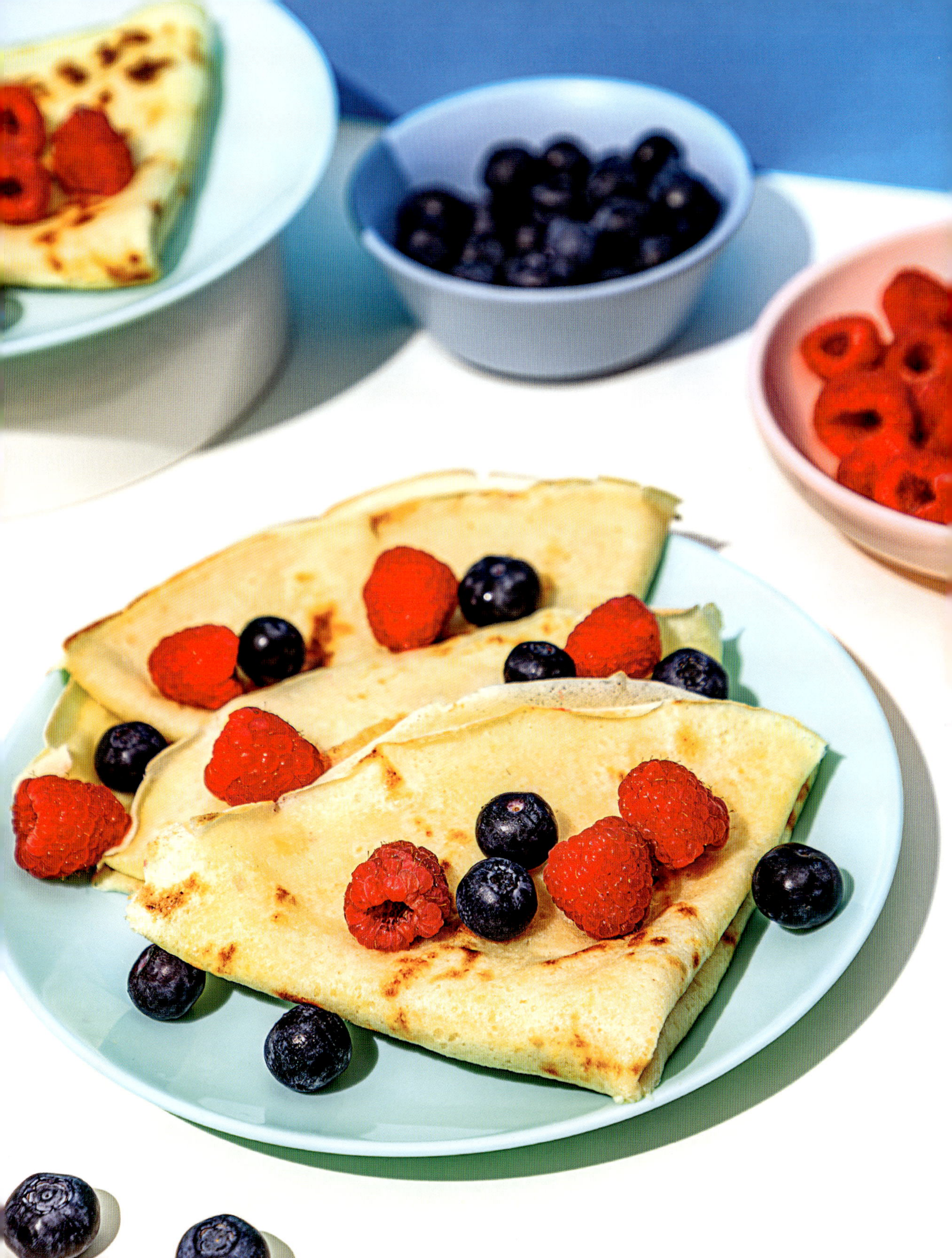

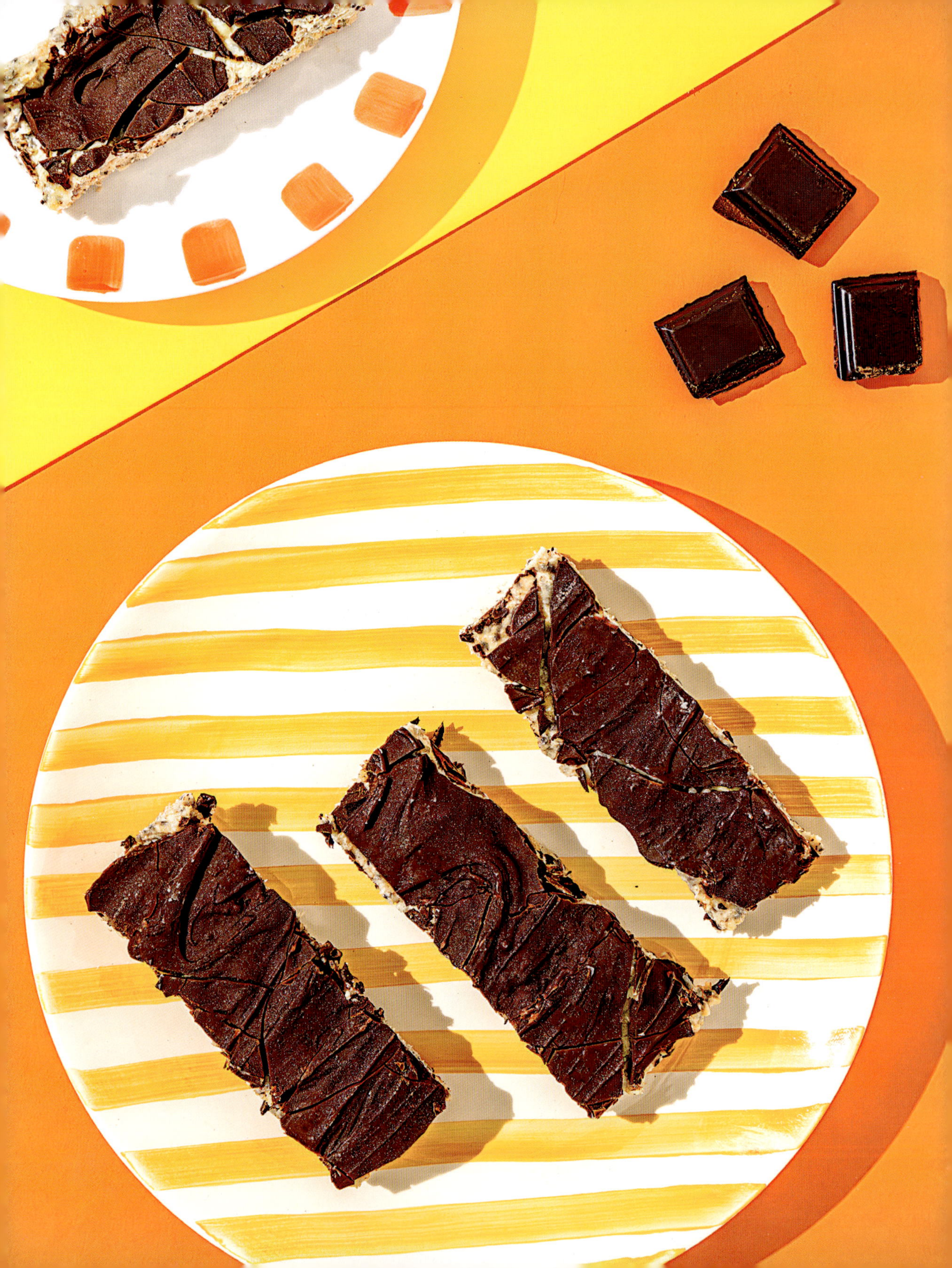

# ALMOND-CHOCOLATE PROTEIN BARS

- FOR 4 PEOPLE
- PREP/COOK TIME: 10 MIN
- REST TIME: 40 MIN IN THE FRIDGE
- ALL SEASONS

1 cup (100 grams) **oats**
¼ cup (60 milliliters) **almond butter**
¼ cup (60 milliliters) **maple syrup**
3 tablespoons (30 grams) **chia seeds**
2 tablespoons (30 grams) **vegan vanilla protein powder**
½ cup (90 grams) **dark chocolate**, coarsely chopped

**1.** In a blender, add all ingredients except the dark chocolate. Blend everything together until the dough holds together when you compact it. You can adjust the texture with a little soy milk if needed.

**2.** Place a sheet of baking paper in the bottom of a square pan and add the dough, spreading it gently with your hands so that it holds together well and the thickness is generally even.

**3.** Place the dough in the freezer for 15 to 20 minutes to allow it to harden. Meanwhile, melt the dark chocolate in a bain-marie.

**4.** Pour the dark chocolate on top and put the mold back in the freezer, again for about 20 minutes.

**5.** When everything is solidified, remove from the pan and cut into bars the size of your choice.

FOR 100 G

| protein: **16.5 g** | carbohydrates: **46.8 g** | lipids: **21 g** |
|---|---|---|

PER PORTION (90 G)

| protein: **14.9 g** | carbohydrates: **42.1 g** | lipids: **18.9 g** |
|---|---|---|

# LUNCH

- FOR 1 PERSON
- PREP TIME: 20 MIN
- SEASON: SUMMER

# "TUNA" SANDWICH

½ (15½-ounce) can (180 grams) **chickpeas**, drained and rinsed
¼ cup **avocado mayonnaise**
1 stalk **celery**, finely chopped
2 sprigs **fresh dill**, finely chopped
**juice of ½ lemon**
2 **sheets seaweed**, finely chopped
2 tablespoons **nutritional yeast**
1 tablespoon **tomato paste**
**salt** and **pepper**, to taste
1 **French multigrain baguette**
1 **tomato**, sliced
4 **cornichons**, cut in strips
some **lettuce**

**1.** In a bowl, mash the chickpeas with a fork.

**2.** Add the avocado mayonnaise, celery, dill, lemon juice, seaweed sheets, nutritional yeast, and tomato paste. Mix all ingredients well.

**3.** Season with salt and pepper to taste. Add more lemon juice if necessary to adjust acidity.

**4.** Cut your baguette into two equal halves, then cut each half open to make two sandwiches.

**5.** Spread prepared "tuna" evenly and generously on one side of each sandwich.

**6.** Add a few slices of tomatoes, some cornichon strips, some lettuce, and put the other side of the sandwich on top.

## Tip

For a pretty look or if you're on the go, wrap your sandwiches in craft paper and tie with string.

FOR 100 G

| protein: **6.4 g** | carbohydrates: **23 g** | lipids: **6.7 g** |
|---|---|---|

PER PORTION (270 G)

| protein: **17.3 g** | carbohydrates: **62.1 g** | lipids: **18.1 g** |
|---|---|---|

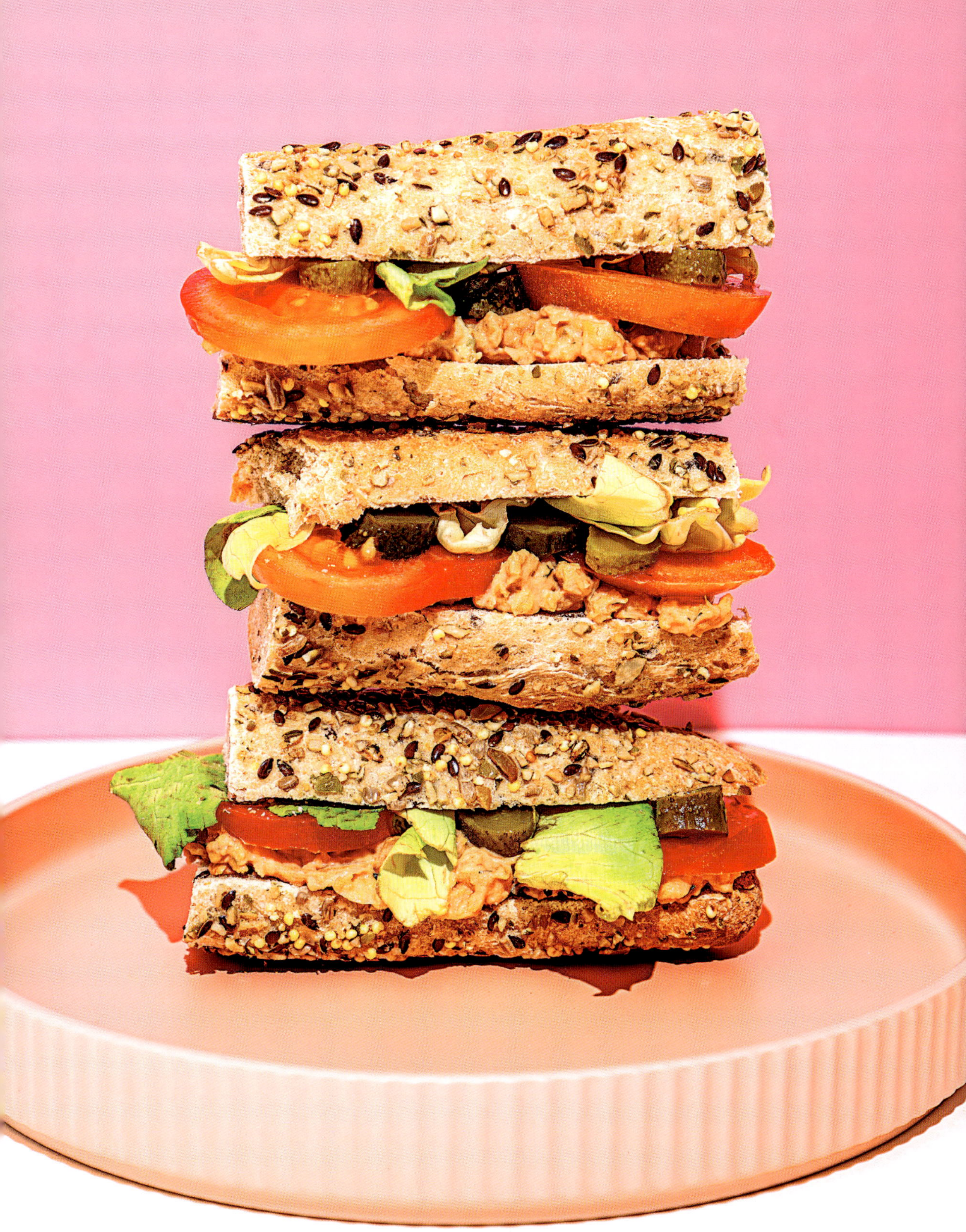

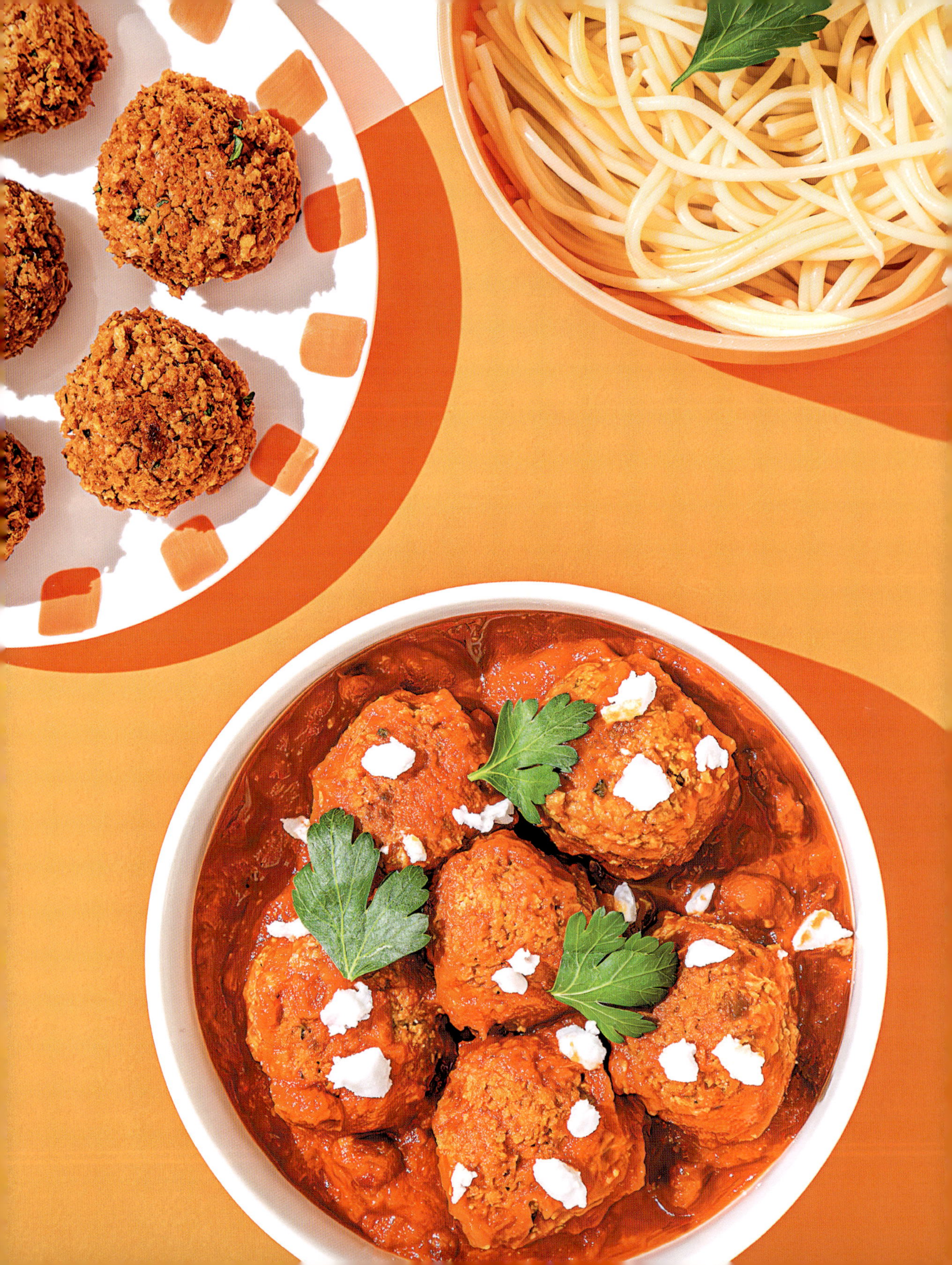

# SOY MEATBALLS WITH SAUCE

- FOR 3 PEOPLE (APPROXIMATELY 15 MEATBALLS)
- PREP/COOK TIME: 40 MIN
- REST TIME: 15 MIN
- ALL SEASONS

**FOR THE MEATBALLS**

1 cup (150 grams) **TSP**
1 **onion**, peeled
2 tablespoons **olive oil**
1 teaspoon **brown sugar**
1 teaspoon **ground smoked paprika**
some **fresh parsley**, chopped
1 teaspoon **garlic powder**
2 teaspoons **whole wheat flour**

**FOR THE SAUCE**

1¼ cups (300 grams) **tomato sauce**
2 tablespoons **kidney beans**, drained and rinsed
1 teaspoon **garlic powder**
a drizzle of **olive oil**
a pinch of **sugar**
a pinch **of salt** and **pepper**

**TO SERVE**

**fresh parsley**
**plant-based "feta"**

**1.** Pour boiling water over the textured soy protein (TSP) in a bowl and let it soak for 10 to 15 minutes. Once rehydrated, drain and squeeze to remove the excess water.

**2.** While the TSP is resting, prepare the onion. Slice it, then caramelize it in a pan with 1 tablespoon of olive oil over low heat. Add the sugar when the onion is translucent. Stir regularly to prevent burning, until golden brown.

**3.** In a blender, mix the rehydrated TSP, caramelized onion, ground smoked paprika, chopped fresh parsley, garlic powder, and remaining olive oil until smooth and until obtaining a fairly consistent texture. Transfer the mixture to a large bowl and add the flour. Knead the mixture until the flour is well incorporated. If the mixture is too sticky, add a little more flour. Shape small balls, about ¾ inch in diameter, with your hands.

**4.** In an oven on grill mode or in an air fryer, place the meatballs on baking paper, taking care not to crowd them so that they brown evenly. Cook them for about 15 minutes, turning them halfway through cooking.

**5.** While the meatballs are cooking, pour the tomato sauce into a pan adding the kidney beans over medium heat. Add the garlic powder, olive oil, and sugar. Adjust the seasoning with salt and pepper to taste. When the meatballs are ready, place them in the tomato sauce. Let simmer for 5 minutes.

**6.** When serving, decorate the meatballs with a few fresh parsley leaves and crumble a little plant-based "feta" on top to add a touch of freshness.

FOR 100 G

| protein: **11.8 g** | carbohydrates: **10.8 g** | lipids: **3.2 g** |
|---|---|---|

PER PORTION (200 G)

| protein: **23.6 g** | carbohydrates: **21.6 g** | lipids: **6.4 g** |
|---|---|---|

- FOR 4 PEOPLE
- PREP/COOK TIME: 40 MIN
- REST TIME: 15 MIN
- WINTER

# CAULIFLOWER PIZZA WITH SOY BOLOGNESE

**FOR THE PIZZA DOUGH**

1 small **cauliflower**
1¼ cups (100 grams) **chickpea flour**
⅓ cup (100 grams) **soy "yogurt"**
**salt** and **pepper**, to taste

**FOR THE SOY BOLOGNESE**

⅔ cups (100 grams) **TSP**
1 **onion**, peeled
1 **carrot**
1 tablespoon **olive oil**
2 tablespoons **soy sauce**
1 teaspoon **herbes de provence**
1 cup (200 grams) **tomato sauce**

**FOR THE TOPPING**

2 ounces (50 grams) **white mushrooms,** sliced
a few **black olives**
½ cup (50 grams) **plant-based grated "cheese"** (optional)
a handful of **arugula**

**1.** Preheat the oven to 400°F. Then wash and cut the cauliflower into pieces before blending as finely as possible. Squeeze the cauliflower semolina in a clean tea towel to remove the excess water.

**2.** In a large bowl, mix the drained cauliflower semolina, chickpea flour, soy "yogurt," salt, and pepper. Knead well until you obtain a smooth dough. If it is too sticky, add a little chickpea flour.

**3.** Spread the dough with your hands on the baking sheet covered with baking paper. Bake for 20 to 30 minutes, then take the dough out of the oven without turning it off—we'll use it again!

**4.** While the dough is pre-cooking, prepare the Soy Bolognese. Soak the TSP by placing it in a bowl and covering it with boiling water for 10 to 15 minutes. Once rehydrated, drain and squeeze gently to remove the excess water.

**5.** Meanwhile, cook the finely chopped onion and carrot in a pan with 1 tablespoon of olive oil, until onions are translucent, and carrots are softened. Add the TSP, mix well, then deglaze with soy sauce, and add the herbes of provence and the tomato sauce.

**6.** Spread the Soy Bolognese on the dough. Sprinkle with sliced white mushrooms and black olives. You can also add some plant-based grated "cheese."

**7.** Return to the oven for 10 to 15 minutes until the mushrooms are cooked and the "cheese" melted. When coming out of the oven, let cool slightly and place a small handful of arugula on top.

FOR 100 G

| protein: **8.4 g** | carbohydrates: **12.9 g** | lipids: **1.3 g** |
|---|---|---|

PER PORTION (400 G)

| protein: **33.6 g** | carbohydrates: **51.6 g** | lipids: **5.2 g** |
|---|---|---|

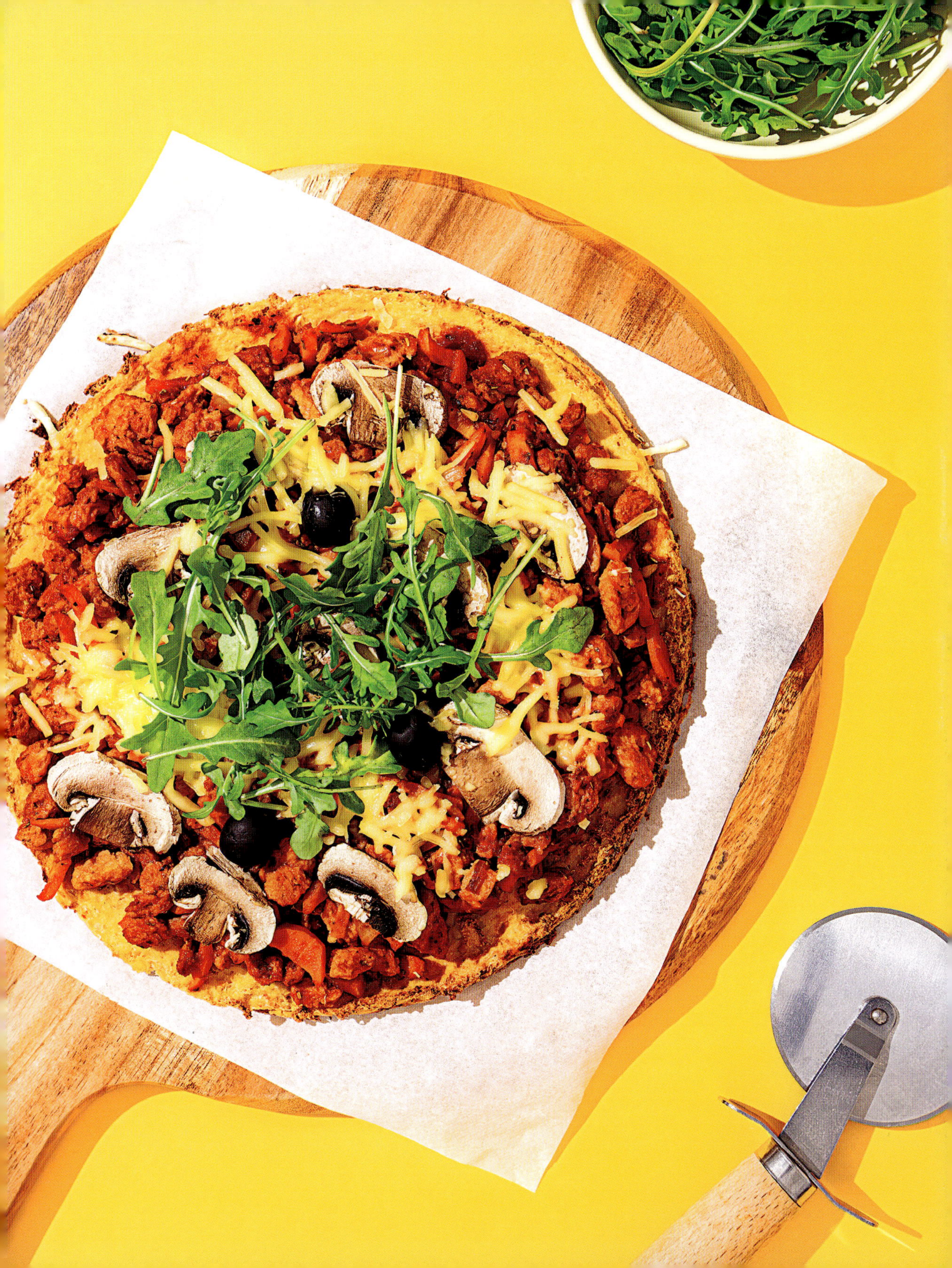

- FOR 2 PEOPLE
- PREP TIME: 35 MIN
- REST: 20 MIN
- ALL SEASONS

# SPRING ROLLS WITH TEMPEH

**FOR THE SPRING ROLLS**

½ pound (250 grams) **tempeh**
1 large **carrot**
¼ **red cabbage**
10 **sheets rice paper**
some **lettuce**, roughly chopped
**mint leaves**

**FOR THE MARINADE**

⅓ cup (15 centiliters) **soy sauce**
2 tablespoons **olive oil**
**ground smoked paprika**, to taste
1 teaspoon **maple syrup**

**FOR THE PEANUT SAUCE**

2 teaspoons **peanut butter**
2 tablespoons **soy sauce**
1 tablespoon **olive oil**

**1.** Start by cutting the tempeh into slices and then into sticks, about ½ inch wide. Then reserve in a large container.

**2.** Prepare the marinade by mixing all the ingredients in a bowl. If necessary, add a little water to increase the quantity. Pour the marinade over the tempeh and let sit for 15 to 20 minutes to allow it to absorb the flavors.

**3.** Meanwhile, prepare the vegetables: Cut the carrot and red cabbage into strips.

**4.** Grill the marinated tempeh sticks in a hot pan for a few minutes on each side, until golden brown. At the end of cooking, deglaze the pan with the remaining marinade to recover the juices and add flavor.

**5.** To soften the rice paper, moisten a sheet in a plate containing water. On a work surface, arrange the ingredients in the center of the rice paper: About 2 tempeh sticks, a little cabbage and carrot, lettuce, and 1 or 2 mint leaves (be careful not to overload the leaf to make rolling easier).

**6.** It's time to make our rolls: Fold over the longest side to enclose all the filling, then fold in the short sides toward the center and roll to form the rolls. Repeat this process to form 10 rolls in total.

**7.** Prepare the peanut sauce by mixing all the ingredients in a bowl. You can adjust the amount and consistency with water, according to your preference.

FOR 100 G

| protein: **8.1 g** | carbohydrates: **12.3 g** | lipids: **9.4 g** |
|---|---|---|

PER PORTION (350 G)

| protein: **28.4 g** | carbohydrates: **43.1 g** | lipids: **32.9 g** |
|---|---|---|

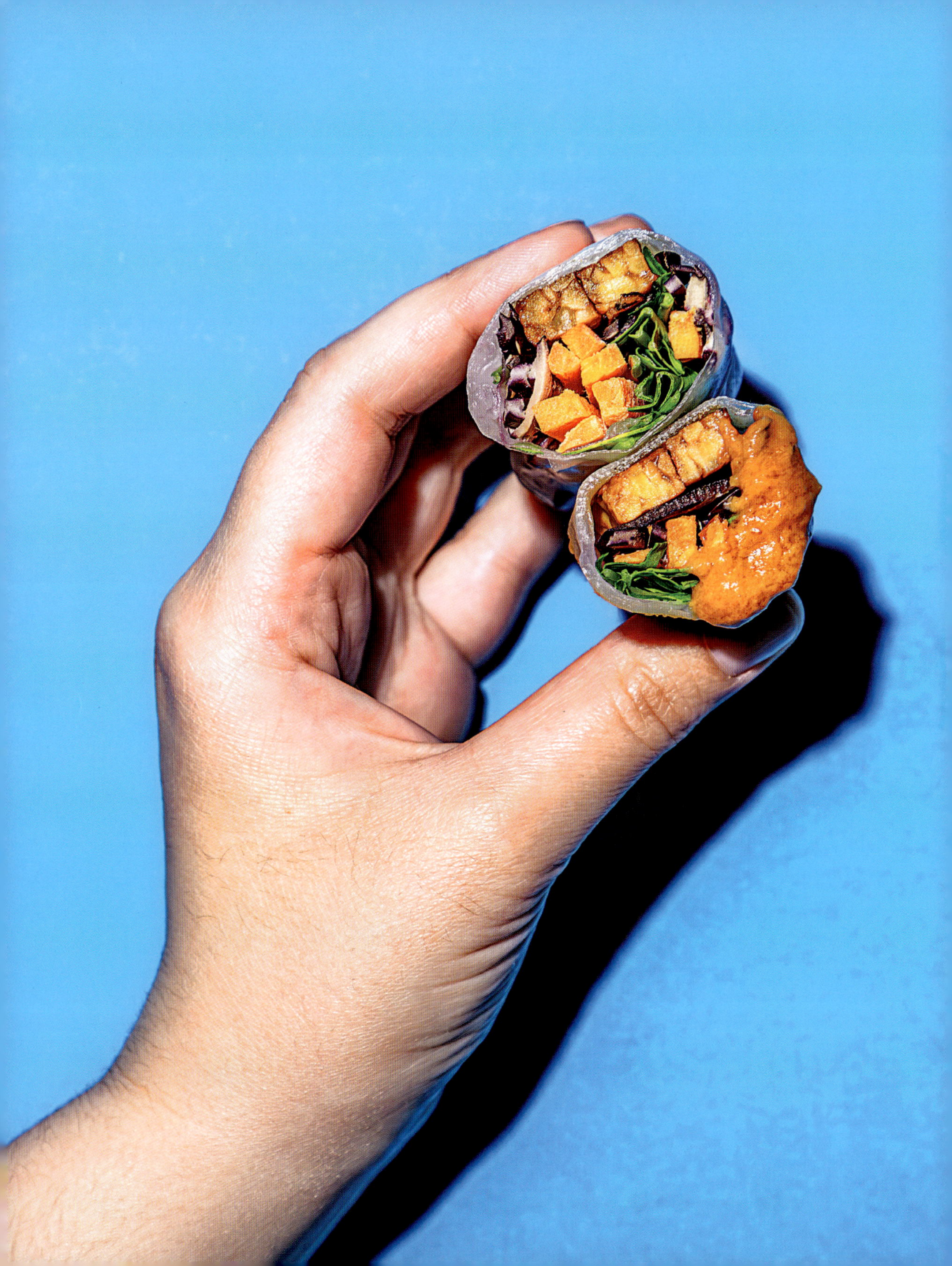

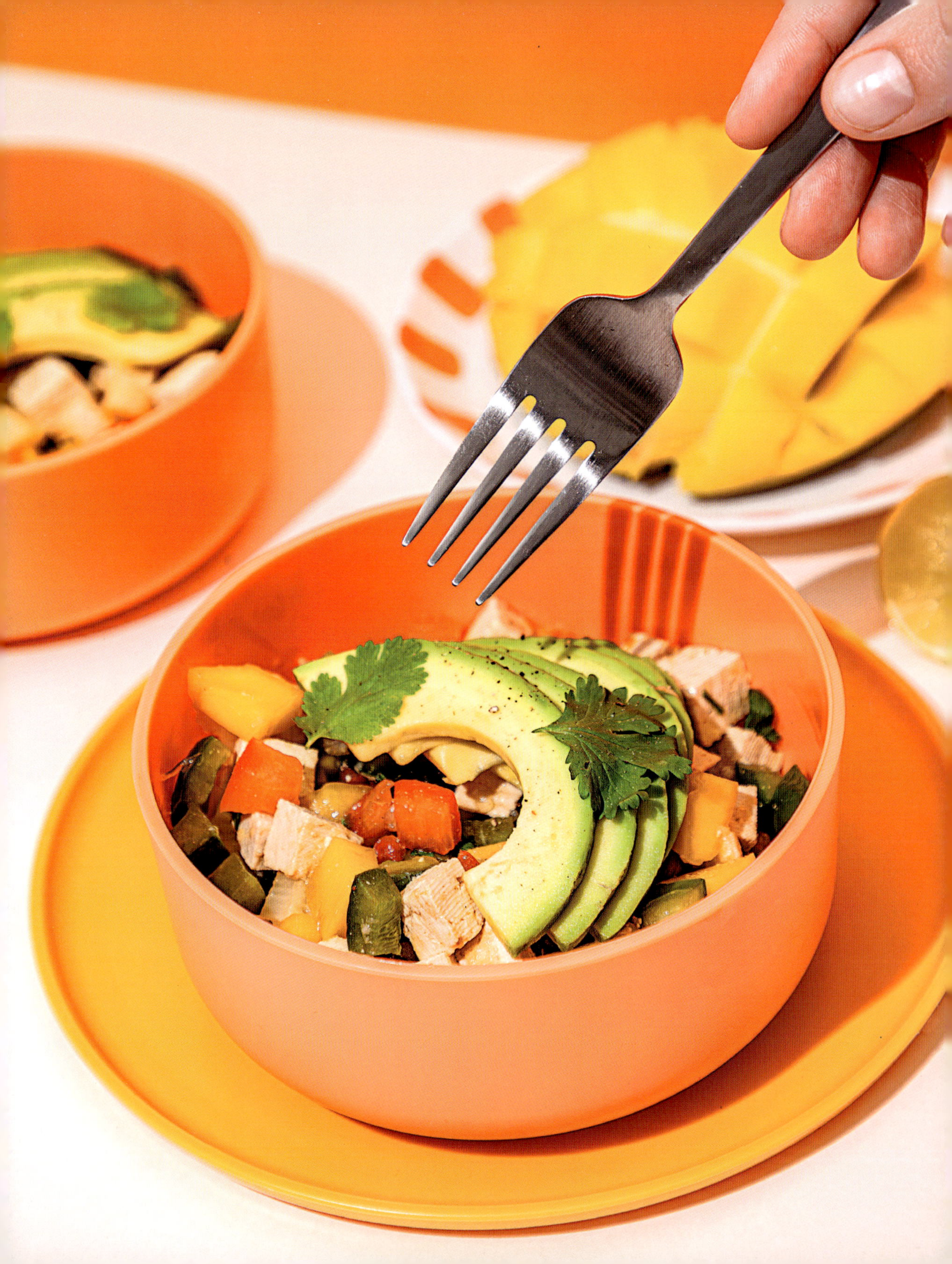

# TOFU CEVICHE WITH PEPPER AND MANGO

- FOR 3 PEOPLE
- PREP/COOK TIME: 45 MIN
- REST TIME: 1 HOUR IN THE FRIDGE
- SUMMER

7 ounces (200 grams) **tofu**
2 **hearts of palm**
1 **tomato**
½ **green pepper**
½ **mango**
½ **red onion**
3 stems **fresh cilantro**, finely chopped
**juice of 2 limes**
2 tablespoons **sweet soy sauce**
2 tablespoons **olive oil**
½ **avocado**
2 stems **dill**, chopped
2 tablespoons **seaweed flakes** or a **sheet** shred into pieces

**1.** Dice the tofu, hearts of palm, tomato, pepper, mango, and red onion into ¼-inch cubes. You can use a mandolin to make cutting vegetables easier.

**2.** In a bowl, mix the tofu and the chopped vegetables and add half of the finely chopped cilantro, lime juice, sweet soy sauce, and olive oil.

**3.** Mix well and let sit in a cool place for at least 1 hour, so that the tofu absorbs the flavors well.

**4.** Arrange in a bowl. Then cut the ½ avocado into thin slices and place them nicely on top with the rest of the chopped fresh cilantro, chopped dill, and seaweed flakes.

## Tips

- You can add a little chili or Tabasco if you like it spicy!
- To avoid browning, cut the avocado right before serving.

FOR 100 G

| protein: **5.1 g** | carbohydrates: **6.3 g** | lipids: **6.3 g** |
|---|---|---|

PER PORTION (300 G)

| protein: **15.1 g** | carbohydrates: **18.7 g** | lipids: **18.7 g** |
|---|---|---|

- FOR 2 PEOPLE (8 DUMPLINGS)
- PREP/COOK TIME: 25 MIN
- WINTER

# RICE PAPER DUMPLINGS WITH TOFU

7 ounces (200 grams) **tofu**
2 stalks **green onions**, finely chopped
1 stalk **celery**, finely chopped
1 **carrot**
2 tablespoons **soy sauce**
16 **sheets rice paper**
1 tablespoon **olive oil**
**salt** and **pepper**, to taste

**1.** In a bowl, crumble the tofu and add the finely chopped green onions and celery, the grated carrot, and the soy sauce. Season with salt and pepper to taste. Mix well. In a frying pan, pour the olive oil and brown everything over medium heat for 5 to 7 minutes, stirring regularly.

**2.** Soak a rice paper sheet in warm water for about 15 seconds, until slightly softened. Remove it from the water and place it on a clean, flat surface.

**3.** Place a spoonful of the stuffing in the center of the softened rice paper. Fold the 4 sides of the rice paper over the stuffing to form a small packet, making sure the stuffing does not leak out.

**4.** Once wrapped in rice paper, wrap the stuffing in another softened rice paper sheet. This will give a crispy finish after cooking.

**5.** Repeat the process with the remaining rice paper sheets and remaining stuffing.

**6.** Once all the dumplings are formed, brown them in a pan with 1 tablespoon of olive oil until golden and crispy.

## Tip

Serve with a little more soy sauce or peanut sauce (see page 66, Spring Rolls with Tempeh).

FOR 100 G

| protein: **9.1 g** | carbohydrates: **17 g** | lipids: **4.1 g** |
|---|---|---|

PER PORTION (270 G)

| protein: **24.6 g** | carbohydrates: **45.9 g** | lipids: **11.1 g** |
|---|---|---|

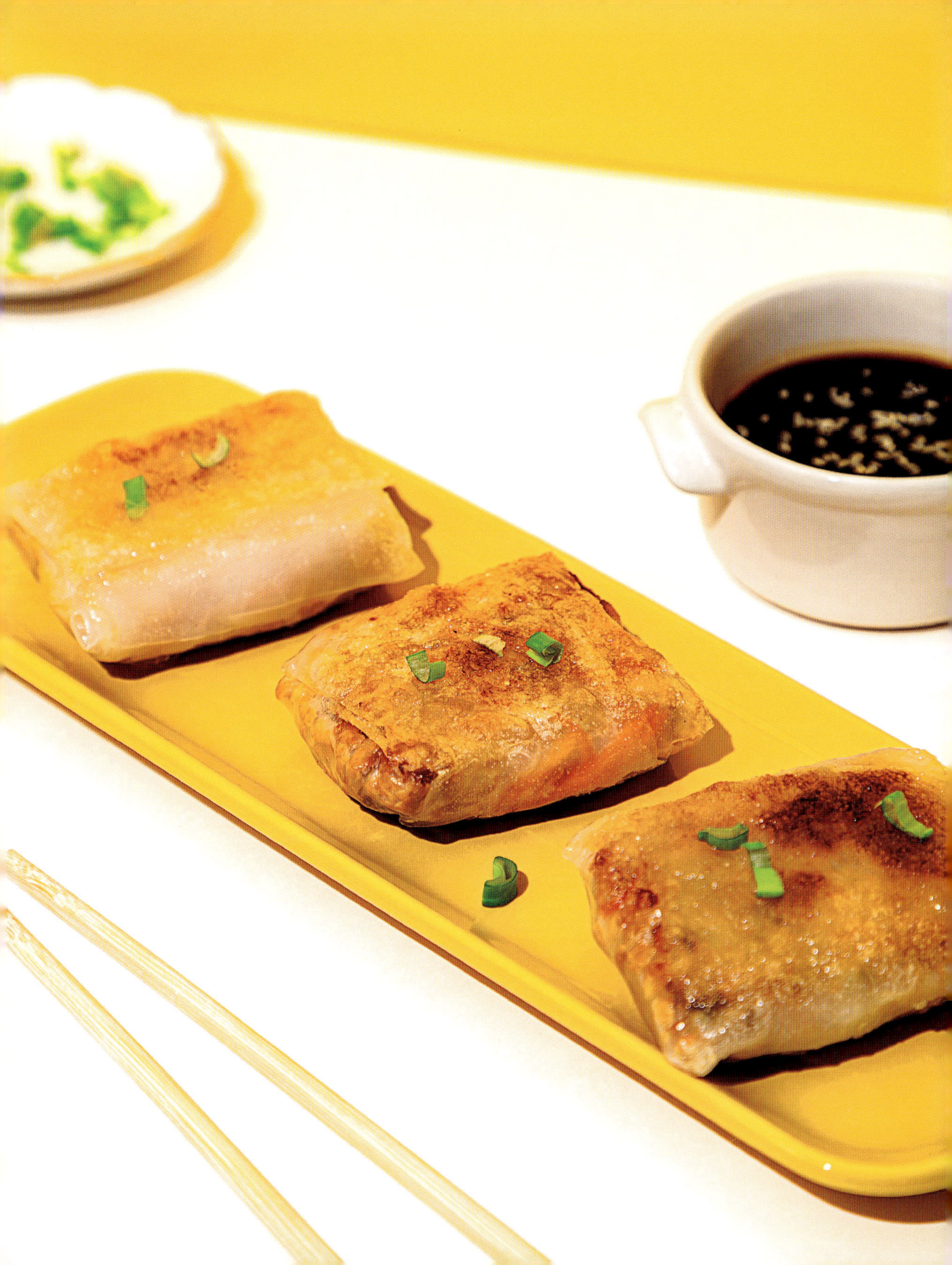

# GREEN BULGUR SALAD

**FOR 2 PEOPLE • PREP/COOK TIME: 25 MIN • REST TIME: 30 MIN IN THE FRIDGE • SUMMER**

**FOR THE SALAD: • 1 cup (200 grams) bulgur • ⅔ cup (100 grams) frozen edamame (soybeans) • ¼ cup (50 grams) pickles • ½ cucumber • 1 green pepper • 2 tablespoons gomashio (Japanese sesame seeds topping)**
**FOR THE SAUCE: • 2 tablespoons miso paste • 2 tablespoons soy sauce • 2 tablespoons nutritional yeast • 1 tablespoon agave syrup • ½ teaspoon wasabi, or more to taste • a few stems fresh cilantro (or fresh parsley)**

**1.** Cook the bulgur according to the package instructions. Then let cool to room temperature. **2.** Cook the edamame in salted boiling water for 5 minutes. Drain and let cool. **3.** Chop the pickles and cut the cucumber and pepper into small cubes. **4.** Add the gomashio. Then mix all ingredients in a large bowl. **5.** In a blender, add all sauce ingredients and blend until you obtain a smooth sauce. Add a little water to adjust the consistency if necessary. **6.** Toss the salad with the dressing and let sit in the refrigerator for at least 30 minutes before serving, to allow the flavors to develop.

| FOR 100 G | | | PER SERVING (380 G) | | |
|---|---|---|---|---|---|
| protein: **5.8 g** | carbohydrates: **23.4 g** | lipids: **2.4 g** | protein: **21.9 g** | carbohydrates: **88.4 g** | lipids: **9 g** |

---

# POTATO SALAD WITH SEITAN

**FOR 4 PEOPLE • PREP/COOK TIME: 30 MIN • ALL SEASONS**

**FOR THE SALAD: • 1¾ cups (400 grams) potatoes • 10½ ounces (300 grams) seitan "sausages" • ½ tablespoon olive oil • ½ cup (100 grams) pickles • ½ red onion**
**FOR THE SAUCE: • ⅓ cup (100 grams) plain plant-based "yogurt" • 3 tablespoons (30 grams) nutritional yeast • 2 tablespoons Dijon mustard • 2 tablespoons apple cider vinegar • 2 tablespoons maple syrup • 1 cup (20 grams) fresh parsley, chopped • salt and pepper, to taste**

**1.** Cook the potatoes in a pan of salted boiling water until tender but still firm, about 15 to 20 minutes. Drain and let cool slightly. **2.** Meanwhile, cut the seitan "sausages" into slices about ¼ inch thick and brown them in a pan with olive oil until golden brown. **3.** Cut the pickles and red onion into small cubes. **4.** In a large bowl, mix the cooked and diced potatoes with the seitan "sausage" slices, pickles, and red onion. **5.** Prepare the sauce by mixing all the ingredients in a bowl until smooth. Season with salt and pepper. **6.** Pour the dressing over the salad and mix well.

**Tips:** You can use commercial seitan "sausages" (some contain up to 29 grams of protein per 100 grams) or make them yourself by shaping your seitan while cooking (see page 83, Caesar Salad with Homemade Seitan).

| FOR 100 G | | | PER PORTION (400 G) | | |
|---|---|---|---|---|---|
| protein: **11.7 g** | carbohydrates: **12.4 g** | lipids: **2.4 g** | protein: **46.8 g** | carbohydrates: **49.6 g** | lipids: **9.7 g** |

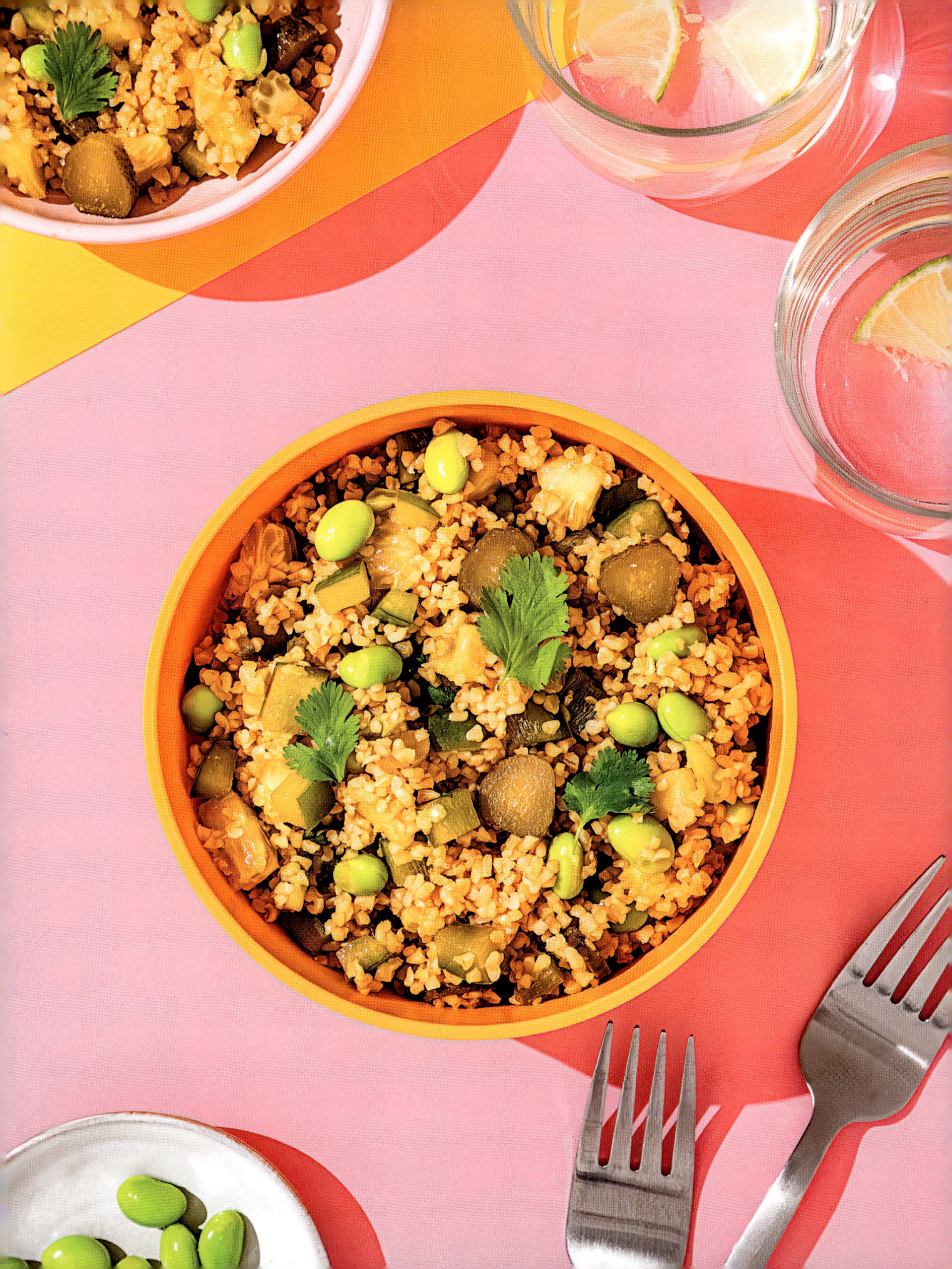

- FOR 2 PEOPLE (4 TRIANGLES)
- PREP/COOK TIME: 25 MIN
- ALL SEASONS

# CLUB SANDWICH WITH GRILLED TEMPEH AND RED CABBAGE

**FOR THE GRILLED TEMPEH**

7 ounces (200 grams) **tempeh**
1 tablespoon **olive oil**
1 teaspoon **ground smoked paprika**
1 teaspoon **garlic powder**
1 tablespoon **sweet soy sauce**

**FOR THE PEANUT SAUCE**

2 teaspoons **peanut butter**
1 teaspoon **mustard**
**juice of ¼ lemon**
1 tablespoon **olive oil**
1 tablespoon **sweet soy sauce**
2 teaspoons **nutritional yeast**
**pepper**

**TO SERVE**

4 slices **sandwich bread**
some **lettuce**
¼ **red cabbage**, finely chopped

**1.** Thinly slice the tempeh and season the slices with ground smoked paprika, garlic powder, and a drizzle of sweet soy sauce. Add the olive oil to a large pan and brown the tempeh until well grilled on both sides. Reserve.

**2.** While the tempeh is grilling, mix all peanut sauce ingredients in a bowl until smooth. Reserve.

**3.** Lightly toast the slices of bread.

**4.** Meanwhile, prepare the green salad by washing it and cutting it into large pieces, then finely chopping the quarter of red cabbage.

**5.** Once the bread is toasted, assemble the sandwiches: Spread a generous layer of peanut sauce on a slice of bread, arrange some lettuce and a handful of shredded red cabbage on top, then add the slices of grilled tempeh. Close the sandwich with another slice of bread.

**6.** Cut each sandwich in half diagonally to make 4 triangles.

FOR 100 G

| protein: **10.3 g** | carbohydrates: **16 g** | lipids: **7.5 g** |
|---|---|---|

PER SERVING (290 G)

| protein: **30.3 g** | carbohydrates: **46.9 g** | lipids: **21.9 g** |
|---|---|---|

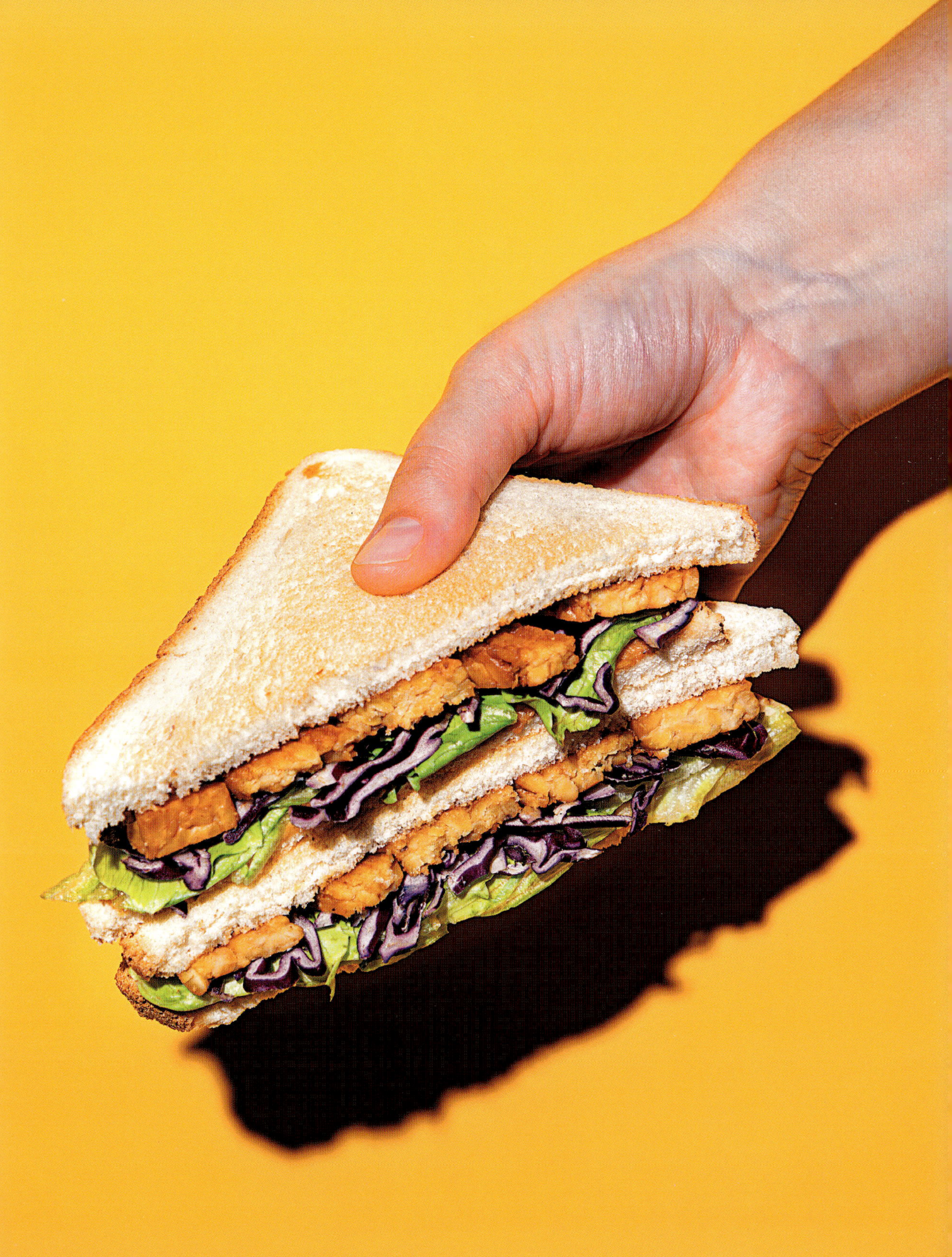

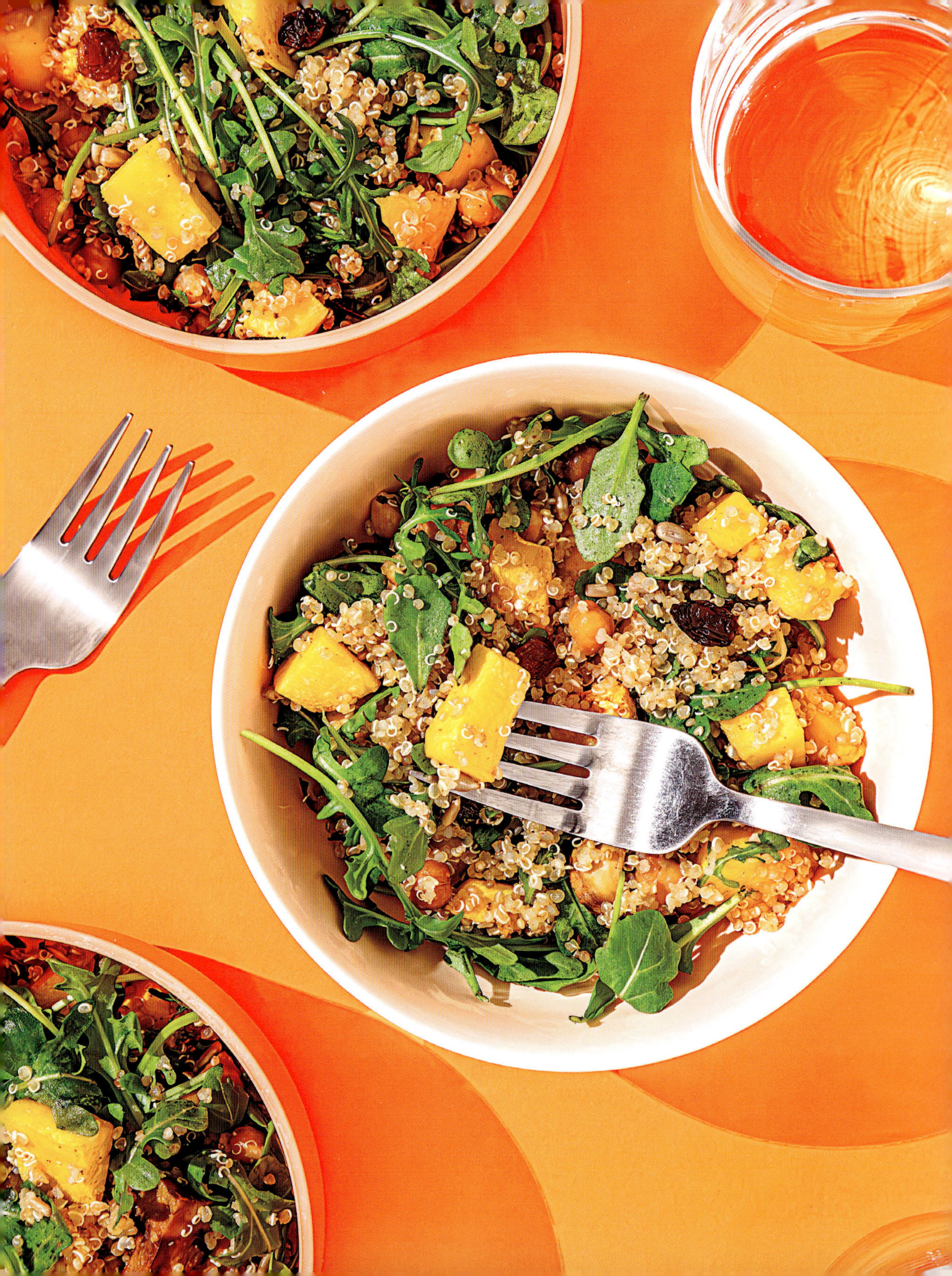

# WINTER SALAD WITH QUINOA AND BUTTERNUT SQUASH

**FOR 4 PEOPLE • PREP/COOK TIME: 30 MIN • WINTER**

**• 1½ cups (250 grams) quinoa • ¼ butternut squash, cut into cubes • 7 ounces (200 grams) white mushrooms, quartered • 1 (15½-ounce) can (400 grams) chickpeas, drained and rinsed • 1 onion • 3 tablespoons olive oil • 2 teaspoons garlic powder • 2 teaspoons ground smoked paprika, to taste • 4 handfuls of arugula • a handful of sunflower seeds • 1 handful of raisins • juice of ½ lemon • salt and pepper, to taste**

**1.** Preheat the oven to 400°F. **2.** Rinse the quinoa under cold water, then cook it according to the instructions on the package. **3.** Prepare the vegetables: Place the butternut squash cubes, quartered white mushrooms, chickpeas, and finely chopped onion on a baking sheet covered with parchment paper. **4.** Drizzle the vegetables and chickpeas with olive oil. Season with salt, pepper, garlic powder, and ground smoked paprika. Mix well. **5.** Place in the oven and bake for about 20 to 25 minutes. **6.** Once done, remove from the oven and let cool slightly. **7.** In a large salad bowl, combine cooked quinoa, roasted vegetables, arugula, sunflower seeds, and raisins. **8.** Drizzle the salad with olive oil and lemon juice. Mix well to distribute the flavors evenly. **9.** Taste and adjust seasoning to your preference.

FOR 100 G

| protein: **5.9 g** | carbohydrates: **20.9 g** | lipids: **6.6 g** |
|---|---|---|

PER PORTION (350 G)

| protein: **20.7 g** | carbohydrates: **73.2 g** | lipids: **23.1 g** |
|---|---|---|

---

# LENTIL SALAD AND SMOKED TOFU PACKAGES

**FOR 2 PEOPLE • PREP/COOK TIME : 35 MIN • FALL/WINTER**

**FOR THE SALAD: • 1 cup (200 grams) green lentils • 3½ ounces (100 grams) smoked tofu • 1 tablespoon olive oil • 2 teaspoons ground smoked paprika • 1 shallot • 2 stems fresh dill • ¼ small red cabbage**

**FOR THE TAHINI SAUCE: • 2 tablespoons tahini • juice of ½ lemon • 1 tablespoon apple cider vinegar • 1 tablespoon maple syrup • 2 tablespoons water • salt and pepper, to taste**

**1.** Rinse the lentils in cold water. Then cook them in a saucepan in lightly salted boiling water for about 20 to 25 minutes. Drain and let cool. **2.** Cut a block of smoked tofu into small rectangles. Brown them in a pan with olive oil and ground smoked paprika until golden brown. Reserve. **3.** Finely chop the shallot and dill and thinly slice the red cabbage. **4.** In a large bowl, mix the cooked lentils, smoked tofu strips, shallot, red cabbage, and dill. **5.** Prepare the tahini sauce: Mix all ingredients, add a little water to obtain the desired consistency, and season. Pour the tahini dressing over the lentil salad and toss to coat all ingredients. **6.** Serve the lentil salad with smoked tofu packages garnished with a little extra fresh dill.

FOR 100 G

| protein: **8.6 g** | carbohydrates: **12.6 g** | lipids: **8.2 g** |
|---|---|---|

PER PORTION (350 G)

| protein: **30.1 g** | carbohydrates: **44.1 g** | lipids: **28.7 g** |
|---|---|---|

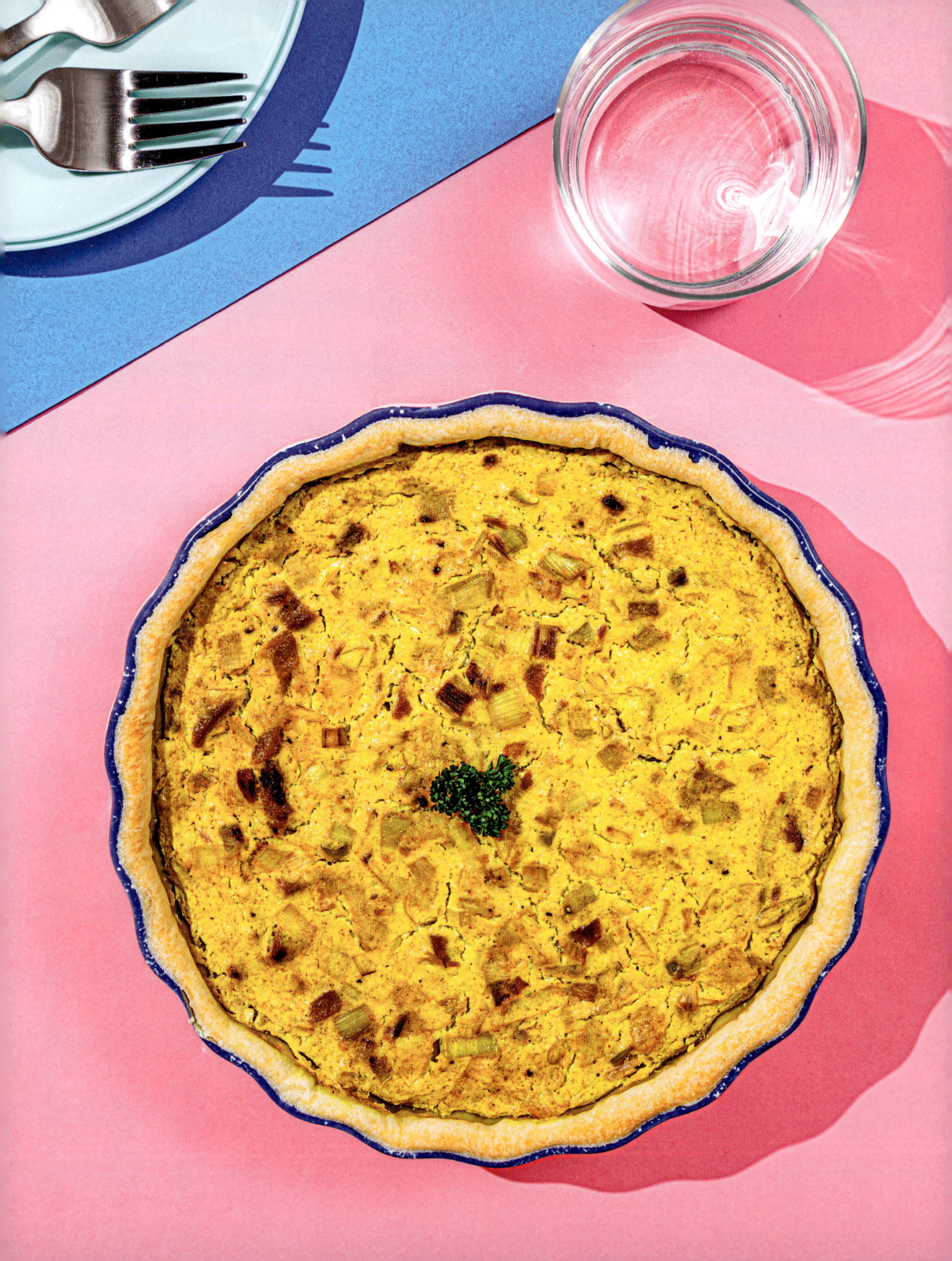

# QUICHE WITH LEEK AND PLANT-BASED "BACON"

- FOR 4 PEOPLE
- PREP/COOK TIME: 45 MIN
- FALL/WINTER

**FOR THE TOPPING**
2 large or 3 small **leeks**
1 **onion**
a drizzle of **olive oil**
½ pound (250 grams) **plant-based "bacon"**

**FOR THE FILLING**
10½ ounces (300 grams) **soft tofu**
2 teaspoons (10 centiliters) **soy cooking cream**
2 teaspoons **ground turmeric**
1 tablespoon **olive oil**
1 tablespoon **soy sauce**
**salt** and **pepper**

**FOR THE BASE**
1 **plant-based puff pastry** (without butter)
1 teaspoon **plant butter**, unsalted
2 tablespoons **mustard**

**1.** Preheat the oven to 350°F.

**2.** Finely chop the leeks and onion. Brown them in a pan with a drizzle of olive oil over medium heat for about 10 minutes, stirring regularly until tender and lightly browned. Reserve.

**3.** In the same pan, cook the plant-based "bacon" until golden and crispy. Reserve.

**4.** Prepare the mixture by combining all the ingredients until you obtain a smooth and creamy texture. Season with salt and pepper to taste. Add the leek and plant-based "bacon" mixture and combine.

**5.** Place the puff pastry in a pie dish previously greased with plant butter. Spread the mustard evenly over the bottom of the tart and pour in the leek and plant-based "bacon" mixture.

**6.** Place the quiche in the preheated oven and bake for 30 to 35 minutes, or until the pastry is golden and crispy.

**7.** Once cooked, let cool for a few minutes before cutting and serving.

FOR 100 G

| protein: **5.2 g** | carbohydrates: **11.7 g** | lipids: **8.3 g** |
|---|---|---|

PER SERVING (330 G)

| protein: **17.2 g** | carbohydrates: **38.6 g** | lipids: **27.4 g** |
|---|---|---|

- FOR 2 PEOPLE
- PREP/COOK TIME: 30 MIN
- SUMMER

# SPICY BLACK BEAN QUESADILLAS

¼ cup **olive oil**
7 ounces (200 grams) **plant-based "chicken" strips**
1 teaspoon **ground cumin**
1 teaspoon **ground paprika**
1 **red onion**
1 **red pepper**
¼ (15-ounce) can (100 grams) **black beans**, drained and rinsed
¼ (15¼-ounce) can (100 grams) **corn**, drained and rinsed
4 whole **wheat or corn tortillas**
1 large **tomato**, diced
1 cup (100 grams) **plant-based grated "cheese"** (optional)
2 stems **fresh cilantro**, chopped
**hot sauce** (optional)
**salt** and **pepper**

**1.** In a frying pan, heat 1 tablespoon of olive oil over medium heat. Add the plant-based "chicken" strips and cook according to the package directions, adding ground cumin, ground paprika, salt, and pepper to season. Once cooked, remove from the pan and set aside.

**2.** In the same pan, add a little more olive oil, if necessary, then sauté the diced red onion and red pepper until tender.

**3.** Add the black beans and drained corn to the pan with the onion and red pepper. Mix well and cook for a few more minutes. Season with salt and pepper to taste.

**4.** Place a tortilla on a clean work surface. Spread some of the vegetable mixture on half of the tortilla. Add ¼ of the previously diced tomato and ¼ of the cooked plant-based "chicken" strips. If desired, sprinkle some plant-based grated "cheese" on top. Fold half of the unfilled tortilla over the other half to form a halfmoon. Repeat the process with the remaining tortillas and remaining ingredients.

**5.** In a large skillet, heat the remaining olive oil over medium heat. Add the quesadillas, 2 at a time if possible, and cook them for about 2 to 3 minutes on each side, until golden and crispy.

**6.** Once cooked, remove the quesadillas from the pan and cut into quarters.

**7.** Top the quesadillas with chopped fresh cilantro and serve warm with hot sauce, if desired.

FOR 100 G

| protein: **4.9 g** | carbohydrates: **10.6 g** | lipids: **1.6 g** |
|---|---|---|

PER SERVING (290 G)

| protein: **25.5 g** | carbohydrates: **55.1 g** | lipids: **8.5 g** |
|---|---|---|

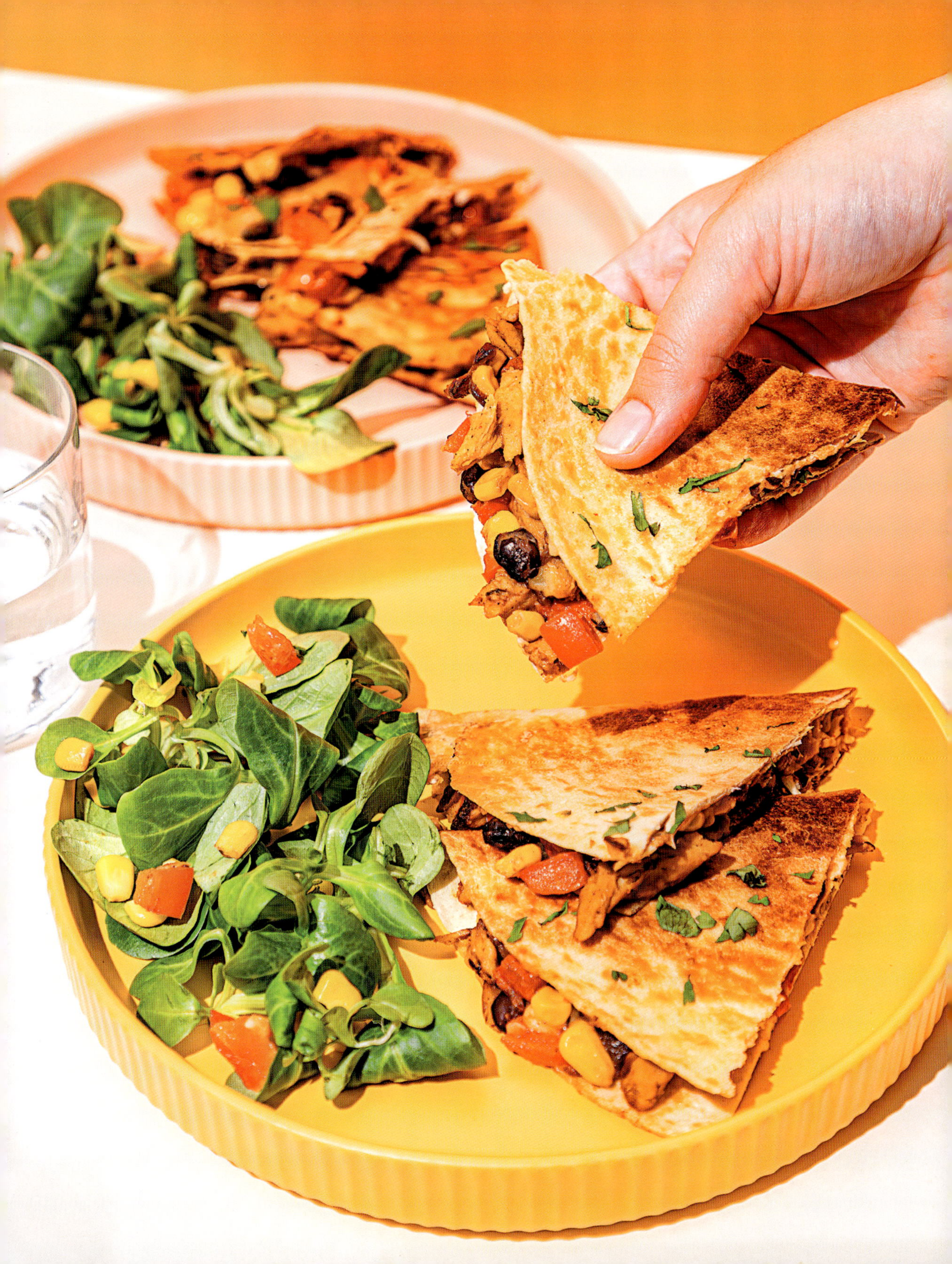

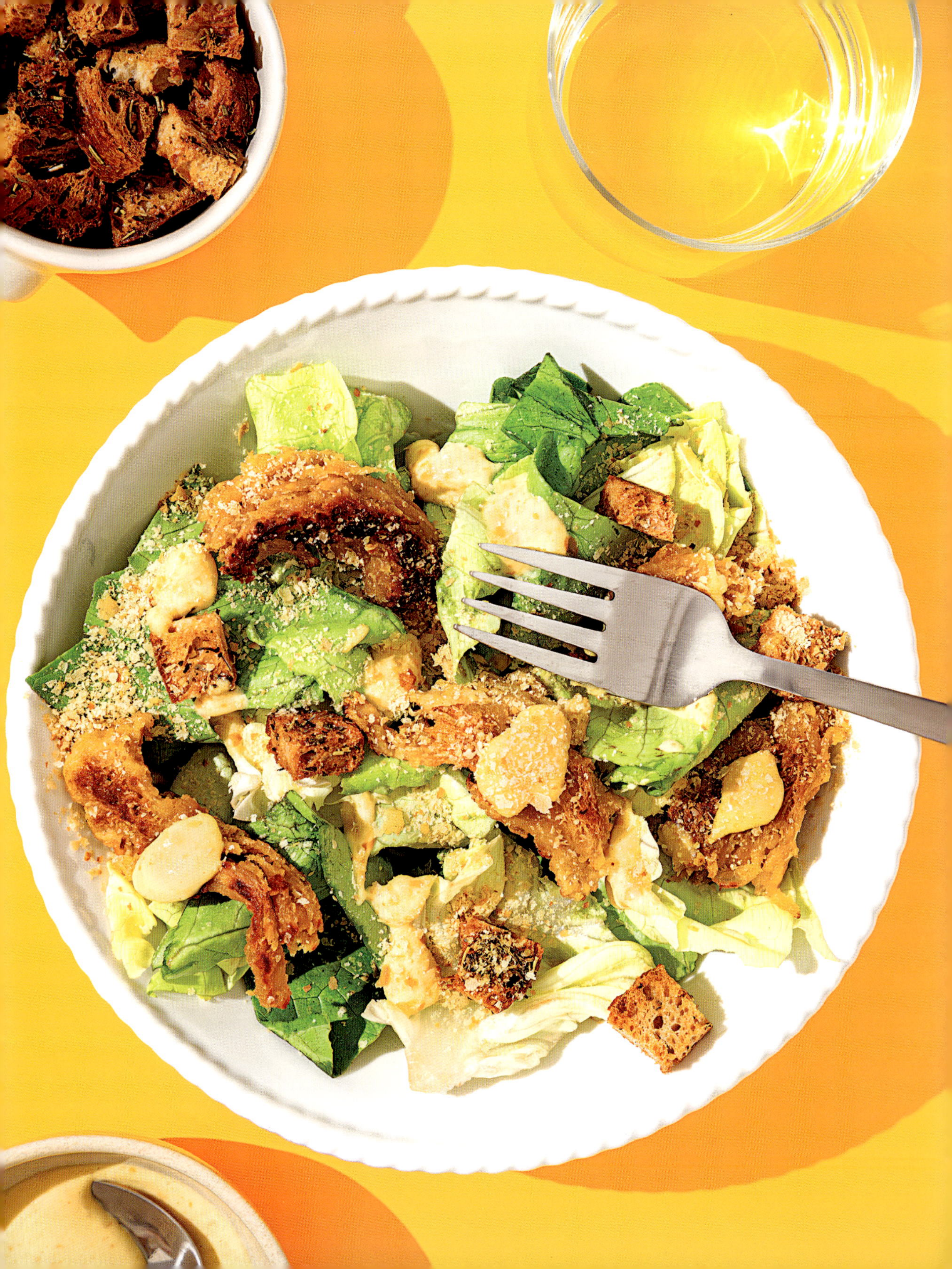

# CAESAR SALAD WITH HOMEMADE SEITAN

- FOR 4 PEOPLE
- PREP/COOK TIME: 1 HOUR 30 MIN
- ALL SEASONS

## STRIPS

**1.** In a blender, mix the chickpeas with water, soy sauce, smoked olive, garlic powder, and mustard until smooth. **2.** Add the flours. Knead the dough for about 10 minutes on a lightly floured work surface, until it is soft and elastic. Form a long sausage with the dough, then tie a simple knot with it to give it a pretzel shape. **3.** In a saucepan, boil water adding a cube of vegetable stock. Add the seitan and cook for 45 minutes over medium heat. **4.** Remove the seitan from the stock and let cool. Then tear it or cut it into thin strips to obtain strips of the desired size. **5.** In a pan with olive oil, grill the seitan strips until they are golden and crispy. Reserve.

## CROUTONS

**1.** Preheat the oven to 350°F. **2.** Cut the slices of bread into cubes. In a bowl, mix the bread cubes with the olive oil, herbes de provence, salt, and pepper, making sure the bread cubes are well coated. **3.** Arrange the bread cubes on a baking sheet and bake for 10 to 15 minutes. Set aside.

## ASSEMBLY

**1.** In a bowl, mix all the ingredients for the plant-based Caesar dressing. **2.** In a large salad bowl, place the romaine lettuce, previously washed and roughly chopped. Add the croutons and spread the grilled strips over the salad, then drizzle generously with the dressing. **3.** Sprinkle with nutritional yeast for added flavor and nutrition.

FOR 100 G

| protein: **14.6 g** | carbohydrates: **8.6 g** | lipids: **7.5 g** |
|---|---|---|

PER PORTION (300 G)

| protein: **43.8 g** | carbohydrates: **25.7 g** | lipids: **22.6 g** |
|---|---|---|

**FOR THE STRIPS**

½ (15½-ounce) can (200 grams) **chickpeas**, drained and rinsed
½ cup (125 milliliters) **water**
2 tablespoons **soy sauce**
1 teaspoon ground **smoked paprika**
1 teaspoon **garlic powder**
1 teaspoon **mustard**
½ cup (75 grams) **whole wheat flour**
1 cup (130 grams) vital **wheat gluten flour**
1 **cube vegetable stock**
2 tablespoons **olive oil**

**FOR THE CROUTONS**

slices of **sourdough bread** or **baguette**
2 tablespoons **olive oil**
1 tablespoon **herbes de provence**
**salt** and **pepper**

**FOR THE PLANT-BASED CAESAR DRESSING**

3 tablespoons **avocado mayonnaise**
2 tablespoons **fresh lemon juice**
1 tablespoon **apple cider vinegar**
1 tablespoon **Dijon mustard**
2 **cloves garlic**, minced
2 tablespoons **nutritional yeast**
**salt** and **black pepper**, to taste

**FOR THE SALAD**

**romaine lettuce**
**nutritional yeast**

- FOR 2 PEOPLE
- PREP/COOK TIME: 50 MIN
- REST TIME: 1 HOUR IN THE FRIDGE
- SUMMER

# SUSHI CAKE WITH TOFU AND EGGPLANT

1½ cups (300 grams) **sushi rice**

**FOR THE VINEGAR**
¼ cup (60 milliliters) **rice vinegar**
1 teaspoon **salt**
2 tablespoons **sugar**

**FOR THE TOFU**
7 ounces (200 grams) **smoked tofu**
2 tablespoons **avocado mayonnaise**
1 teaspoon **ground smoked paprika**

**FOR THE REST OF THE FILLING**
2 **sheets seaweed**
3½ ounces (100 grams) **shiitake mushrooms**, sliced
a drizzle of **olive oil**
1 small **eggplant**
1 tablespoon **sesame seeds**
3 cups (100 grams) **sprouts** (alfalfa)

**TO SERVE**
**soy sauce**

**1.** Start by rinsing your sushi rice under cold water until the water runs clear. Cook it according to the instructions on the package. Meanwhile, prepare the vinegar mixture: Heat the rice vinegar, sugar, and salt in a saucepan over low heat until the sugar and salt are well dissolved. Let cool.

**2.** While the rice is cooking, prepare your tofu: Grate it in a bowl and mix it with the avocado mayonnaise and ground smoked paprika. Reserve.

**3.** Cut the seaweed sheets into strips lengthwise. Brown the sliced shiitake mushrooms in a pan with olive oil until they are tender. Reserve. Cut the eggplant into thin slices lengthwise and then brown them in the same pan in which you cooked the shiitake mushrooms.

**4.** Once the rice is cooked, spread it out on a large dish and drizzle with the vinegar mixture. Mix to coat the rice well with vinegar. Let cool.

**5.** When the rice has cooled, assemble your sushi cake in a cake mold. Start with slices of eggplant at the bottom of the mold (which will be the top of the cake), then a layer of rice, a seaweed sheet, the grated tofu with mayo, a layer of rice, the other seaweed sheet, the shiitake mushrooms, and a last layer of rice. The cake must reach the top of the mold. Press the sushi cake into the mold to compact it. Then place the mold in the refrigerator for at least 1 hour.

**6.** When ready to serve, transfer the sushi cake onto a plate buy putting a plate on top of it, flipping over and then lifting the mold away. Sprinkle with sesame seeds and garnish with sprouts. Carefully cut into slices with a sharp knife and serve with soy sauce.

FOR 100 G

| protein: **7.6 g** | carbohydrates: **20.9 g** | lipids: **7.2 g** |
|---|---|---|

PER PORTION (250 G)

| protein: **19 g** | carbohydrates: **52.3 g** | lipids: **18 g** |
|---|---|---|

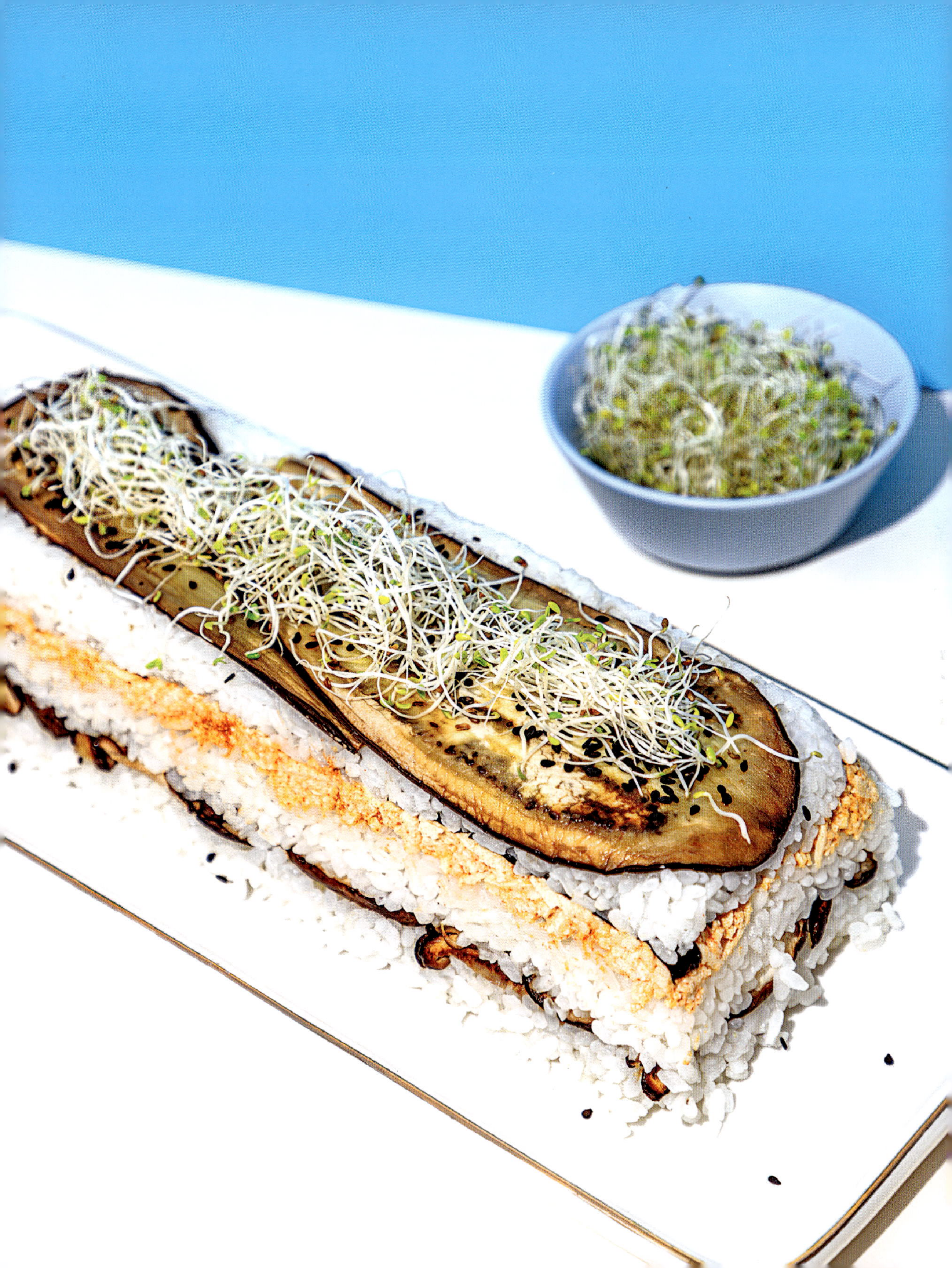

- FOR 2 PEOPLE
- PREP/COOK TIME: 25 MIN
- ALL SEASONS

# BURRITO WITH VEGETABLE SLICES AND COLESLAW

**FOR THE HUMMUS**

½ (15½-ounce) can (200 grams) **chickpeas,** drained and rinsed
2 tablespoons **tahini**
2 tablespoons **olive oil**
1 tablespoon **apple cider vinegar**
**juice of ½ lemon**
a pinch of **sea salt**

**FOR THE COLESLAW**

1 cup (100 grams) **red cabbage**, chopped
1 cup (100 grams) **white cabbage**, chopped
2 tablespoons **olive oil**
**juice of ½ lemon**
a pinch of **sea salt**

**FOR THE BURRITO**

1 **head romaine lettuce**
5 to 6 ounces (150 to 200 grams) **plant-based "chicken" strips** (homemade—see Caesar Salad page 83—or store-bought)
a drizzle of **olive oil**
2 large **whole wheat crepes**, or 2 **corn tortillas**
2 tablespoons **corn**, drained and rinsed

**1.** In a blender, add all the ingredients to prepare the hummus. Blend until smooth. If necessary, add a little water to obtain the desired consistency. Reserve.

**2.** Prepare the coleslaw: Grate the cabbages and season them with oil, salt, and lemon. Reserve.

**3.** Cut the lettuce into strips and brown the plant-based "chicken" slices in a frying pan over medium heat for about 10 minutes with a light drizzle of olive oil. Stir regularly until heated through and lightly browned.

**4.** It's time to assemble the burrito! Place a whole wheat crepe or corn tortilla on a clean surface. In the center of the crepe or tortilla, spread a good portion of the home-made hummus, then add a handful of coleslaw, corn, lettuce, and sautéed plant-based "chicken" strips. Fold the top and bottom of the crepe or tortilla towards the center, then roll it tightly around the filling to form your burrito.

**5.** Finally, grill your burrito in a pan over medium heat for 1 to 2 minutes on each side, or air fry it for about 5 minutes until crispy on the outside.

**6.** All you have to do is bite into it and enjoy!

FOR 100 G

| protein: **10.6 g** | carbohydrates: **23 g** | lipids: **13.6 g** |
|---|---|---|

PER PORTION (300 G)

| protein: **31.9 g** | carbohydrates: **69.1 g** | lipids: **40.7 g** |
|---|---|---|

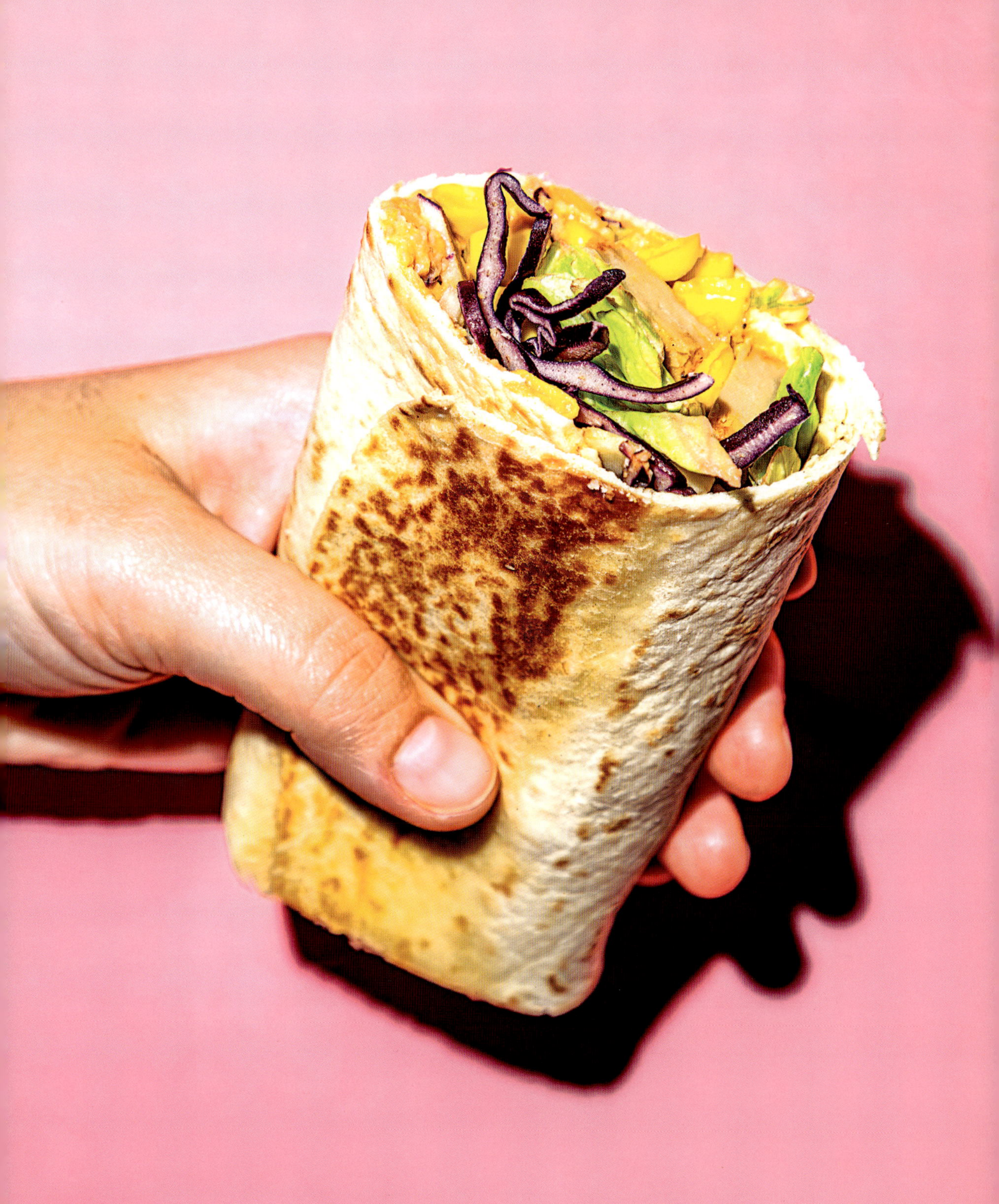

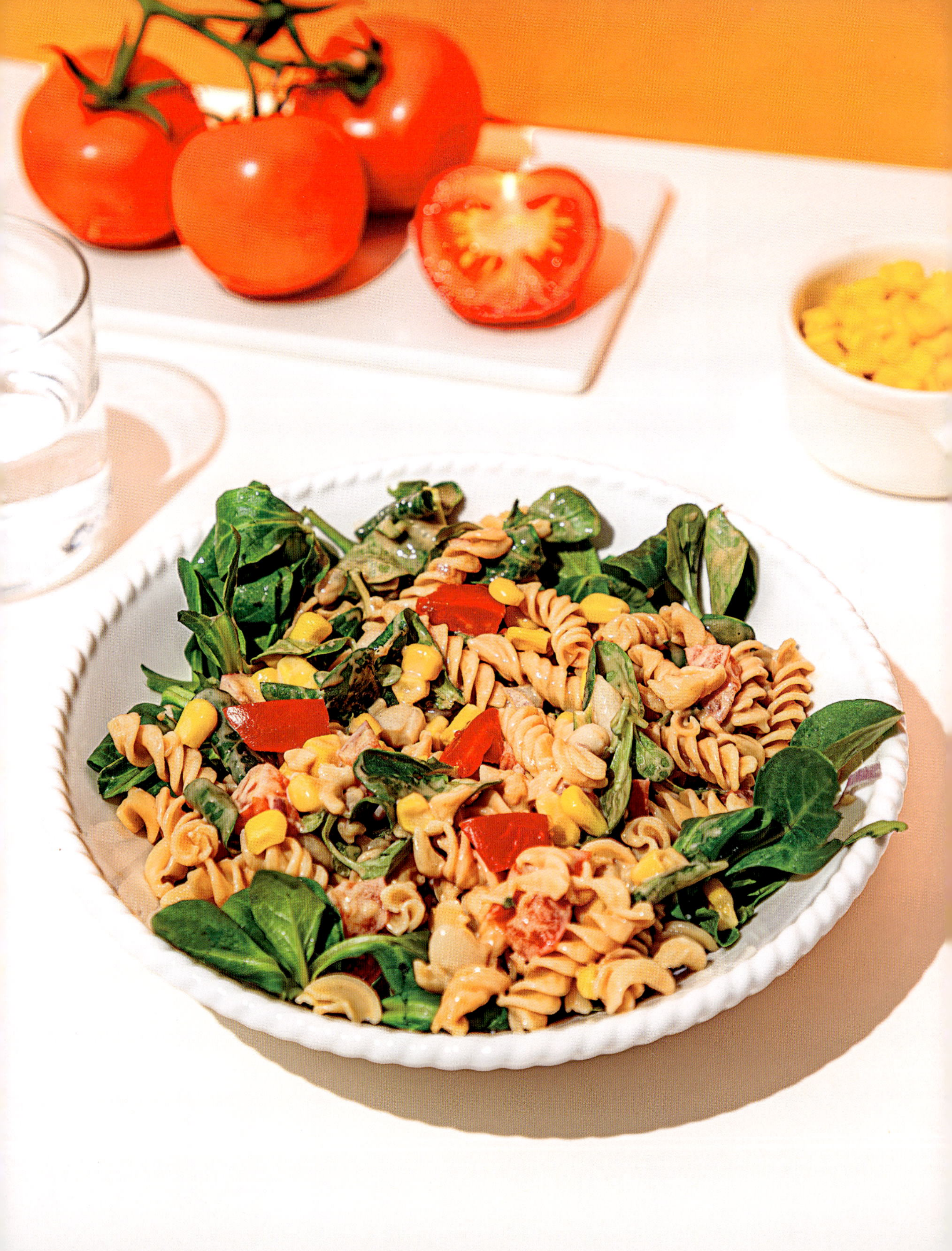

# PASTA SALAD WITH RED LENTILS AND WHITE BEANS

- FOR 4 PEOPLE
- PREP/COOK TIME: 30 MIN
- REST: 30 MIN IN THE FRIDGE
- SUMMER

**FOR THE SALAD**

7 ounces (200 grams) **red lentil pasta**
¼ (15-ounce) can (100 grams) **white beans**, drained and rinsed
3½ ounces (100 grams) **arugula**
approximately ⅓ (15¼-ounce) can (140 grams) **corn**, drained and rinsed
2 **tomatoes**, diced
1 **shallot**, finely chopped

**FOR THE DRESSING**

2 tablespoons **almond butter**
**juice of ½ lemon**
1 tablespoon **balsamic reduction**
1 tablespoon **olive oil**
1 teaspoon **mustard**
**salt** and **pepper**, to taste

**1.** Cook the red lentil pasta according to the instructions on the package. Once cooked, drain and let cool.

**2.** In a large bowl, mix the cooked red lentil pasta, white beans, lettuce, corn, tomatoes, and shallot.

**3.** Prepare the sauce by mixing all ingredients in a small bowl. Dilute with a little water if necessary.

**4.** Pour the dressing over the red lentil pasta salad and mix well to coat all the ingredients.

**5.** Let salad rest in the refrigerator for at least 30 minutes before serving, to allow salad to marinate.

## Tip

If you want to store this salad, serve the lettuce separately, so that it doesn't wilt.

FOR 100 G

| protein: **9.6 g** | carbohydrates: **24.7 g** | lipids: **5.5 g** |
|---|---|---|

PER PORTION (420 G)

| protein: **40.3 g** | carbohydrates: **103.7 g** | lipids: **23.1 g** |
|---|---|---|

# DINNER

# KATSU CURRY

- FOR 2 PEOPLE
- PREP/COOK TIME: 50 MIN
- FALL/WINTER

**FOR THE CURRY**

1 **onion**, chopped
1 tablespoon **olive oil**
2 **cloves garlic**, minced
1 **carrot**
1 **potato**, peeled and diced
1 cup (150 grams) **frozen peas,** thawed
3½ ounces (100 grams) white **mushrooms**, sliced
2 tablespoons **curry powder**
1 tablespoon **soy sauce**
1 cup (200 milliliters) **coconut milk**
½ cup (10 centiliters) **vegetable broth**

**FOR THE KATSU**

7 ounces (200 grams) **firm tofu**
⅓ cup (50 grams) **all-purpose flour**
¼ cup (50 milliliters) **milk alternative** (soy, for example)
½ cup (50 grams) **breadcrumbs**
1 tablespoon **ground paprika**
1 tablespoon **olive oil**

**TO SERVE**

**rice,** cooked, as a side
**salt** and **pepper**, to taste

**1.** In a hot pan, sauté the chopped onion in olive oil until translucent. Then add minced garlic and brown for a few moments. Add carrot and diced potatoes, peas, and sliced mushrooms. Sauté for a few minutes until the vegetables become tender. Add curry powder, deglaze with soy sauce, pour in coconut milk and broth, and simmer until all flavors soak in well. The consistency of the sauce should be thick but flexible. Let reduce over low heat if necessary or, conversely, add a little broth.

**2.** While you keep your curry warm, make the katsu. Start with cutting the block of tofu widthwise to make 2 slices about ½ inch thick.

**3.** In a bowl, mix the flour with the milk alternative to obtain a smooth paste. In another bowl, mix the breadcrumbs with the ground paprika. Dip each slice of tofu in the flour and milk alternative mixture. Then coat them in paprika breadcrumbs to make katsu.

**4.** In a skillet, heat the olive oil over medium heat. Brown the tofu katsu slices on each side until crispy and golden brown.

**5.** When everything is ready, dress half of a deep plate with rice and the other half with the curry. Then cut the slices of tofu katsu and place them on top.

## Tip

You can also buy ready-to-eat plant-based cutlets if you don't have time to prepare the tofu katsu.

FOR 100 G

| protein: **5.1 g** | carbohydrates: **13.6 g** | lipids: **5.9 g** |
|---|---|---|

PER PORTION (400 G)

| protein: **20.5 g** | carbohydrates: **54.5 g** | lipids: **23.8 g** |
|---|---|---|

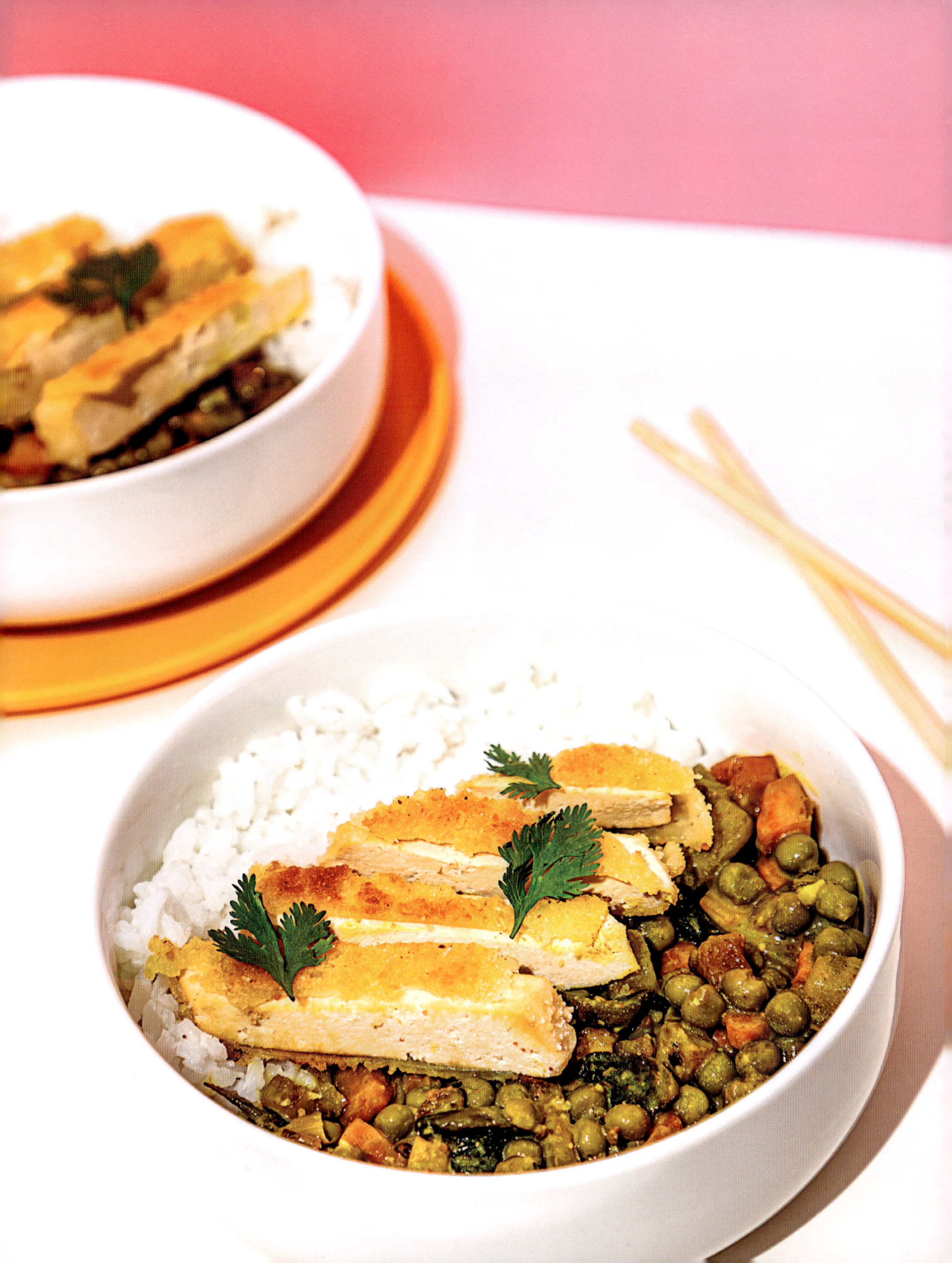

- FOR 2 PEOPLE
- PREP/COOK TIME: 40 MIN
- REST TIME: 10 MIN
- SUMMER, OR ALL SEASON WITHOUT PEPPER AND BROCCOLI

# CARAMELIZED TSP WITH SAUTÉED VEGETABLES

1 cup (150 grams) large **TSP**
3 tablespoons **soy sauce,** divided
2 **onions**
1 piece **fresh ginger** (about ¾ inch)
5 ounces (150 grams) **mushrooms**
1 **red pepper**
1 **small broccoli**
1 tablespoon **olive oil**
1 teaspoon **ground smoked paprika**
1 teaspoon **cumin**
1 teaspoon **ground coriander**
1 tablespoon **sugar**
1 tablespoon **sesame seeds**
a small bunch **fresh cilantro**, chopped

**1.** Start by soaking the TSP in hot water with 1 tablespoon of soy sauce for about 10 minutes. Once rehydrated, drain and squeeze to remove the excess water.

**2.** Meanwhile, chop the onions, grate the piece of fresh ginger, slice the mushrooms, cut the pepper into strips, and cut small florets of broccoli.

**3.** In a frying pan, heat the olive oil over medium heat. Add chopped onions and grated ginger and sauté until golden and fragrant. Add all spices and sugar.

**4.** Then add rehydrated TSP, onions, and ginger to the pan. Let cook for a few minutes over medium heat, stirring from time to time until they brown lightly.

**5.** Add the mushrooms, broccoli, and pepper, and sauté for a few minutes to combine the flavors.

**6.** Deglaze with the remaining soy sauce and cook the vegetables until tender but still crisp.

**7.** Before serving, sprinkle the TSP with sesame seeds and chopped fresh cilantro.

FOR 100 G

| protein: **8.9 g** | carbohydrates: **9.3 g** | lipids: **2.6 g** |
|---|---|---|

PER PORTION (400 G)

| protein: **35.6 g** | carbohydrates: **37.2 g** | lipids: **10.6 g** |
|---|---|---|

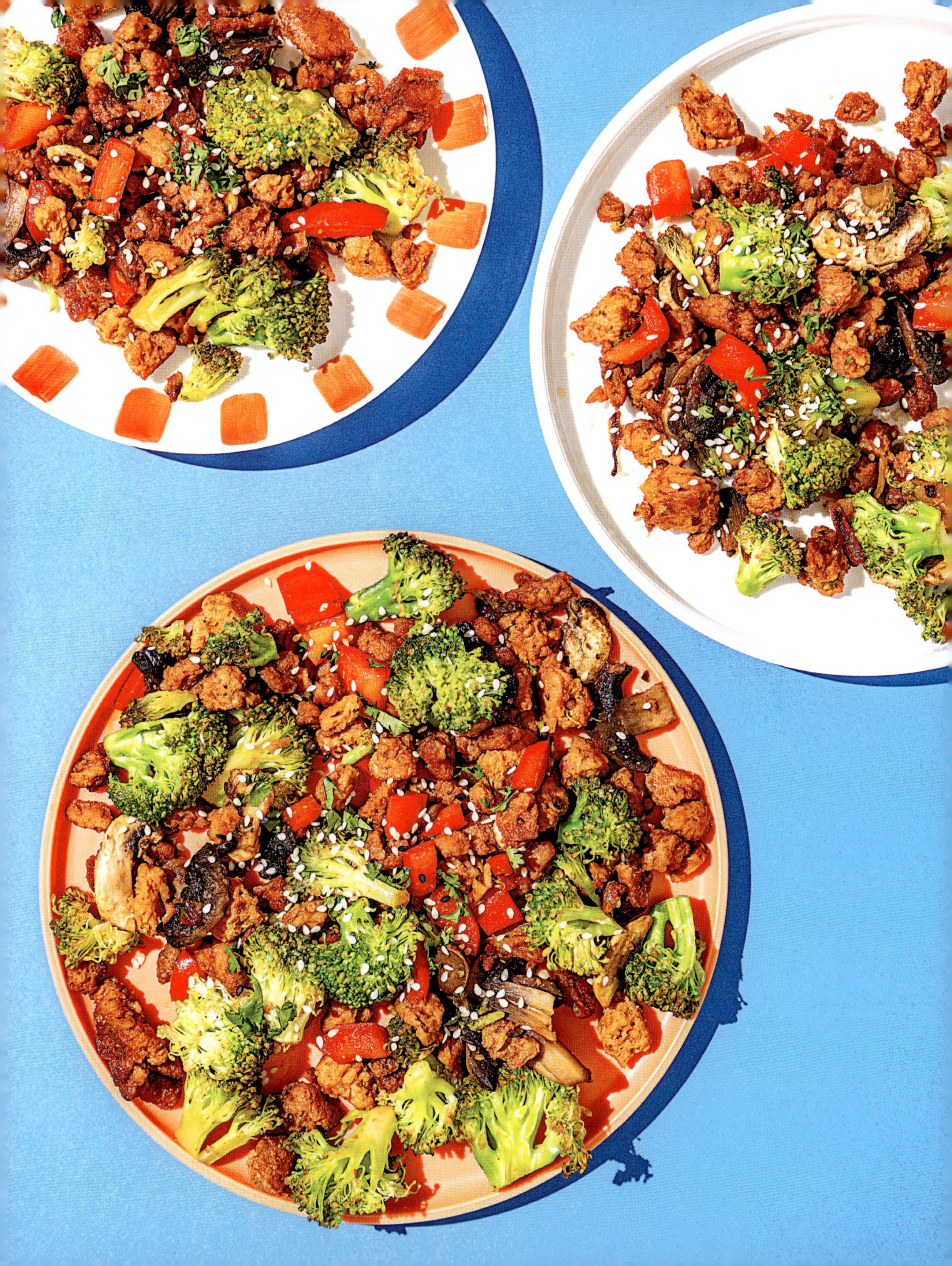

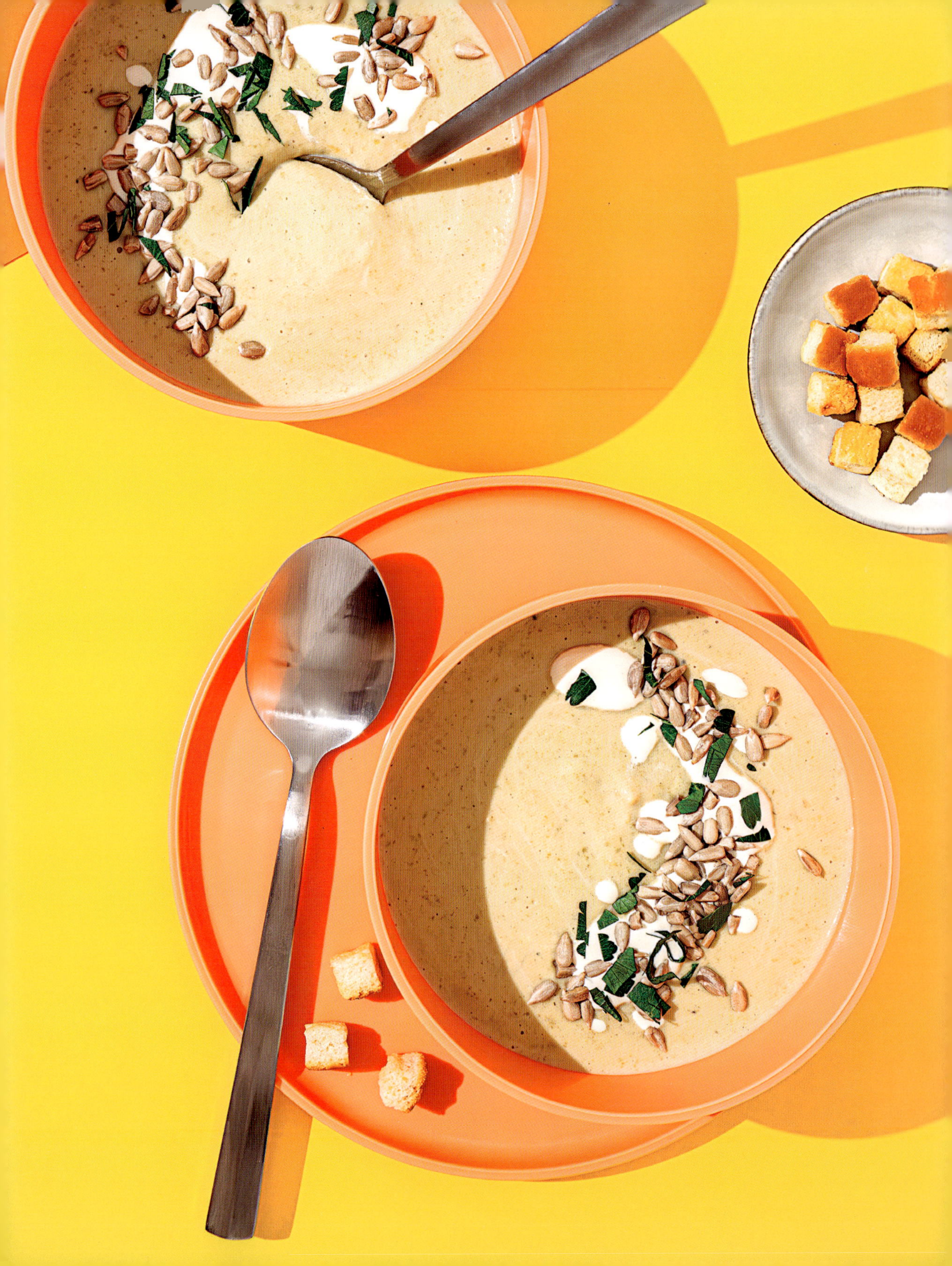

# SPLIT PEA AND ARTICHOKE SOUP

- FOR 3 PEOPLE
- PREP/COOK TIME: 45 MIN
- SPRING/SUMMER

**FOR THE SOUP**
1 cup (250 grams) **split peas**
1 tablespoon **olive oil**
2 **onions**, diced
1 **potato**, cubed
1 **clove garlic**, chopped
5 **artichoke hearts**, quartered
1 cup (20 centiliters) **soy cooking cream**
a pinch of **coarse salt**
4 cups boiling **water**

**FOR THE TOPPING**
¼ cup **soy cooking cream**
a few drops **lemon juice**
1⅓ tablespoons **sunflower seeds**
a few leaves **fresh parsley**, chopped

**1.** Soak the split peas in water for at least 1 hour, ideally overnight.

**2.** In a saucepan, heat 1 tablespoon of olive oil over medium heat. Add the diced onions, cubed potato, and chopped garlic. Brown for about 10 minutes.

**3.** Add the quartered artichoke hearts to the pan. Also add the drained split peas, 4 cups of boiling water, and a pinch of coarse salt. Simmer for about 30 minutes, or until split peas are tender.

**4.** Use an immersion blender to blend the soup until smooth and creamy. Then add the soy cooking cream and mix well.

**5.** To serve, ladle soup into individual bowls. Per bowl, add a drizzle of soy cooking cream a few drops of lemon juice, the sunflower seeds, and chopped fresh parsley on top.

## Tips

- Enjoy with a slice of whole wheat bread or a few croutons (see page 83, Caesar Salad with Homemade Seitan).
- This recipe can be enjoyed as a cold starter.

FOR 100 G

| protein: **6.2 g** | carbohydrates: **19.9 g** | lipids: **3.6 g** |
|---|---|---|

PER PORTION (250 G)

| protein: **15.5 g** | carbohydrates: **49.8 g** | lipids: **9 g** |
|---|---|---|

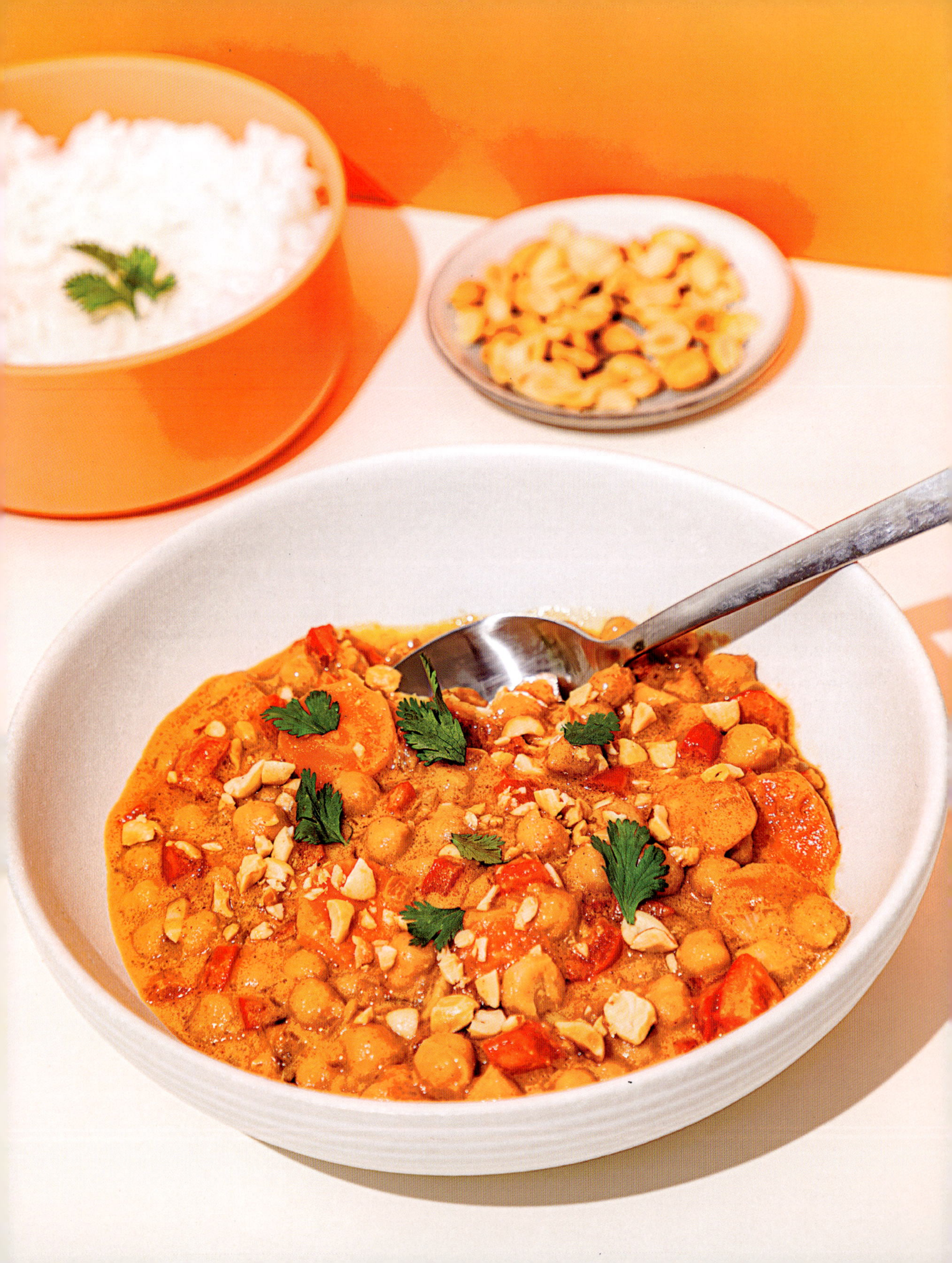

# RED CURRY CHICKPEAS

- FOR 4 PEOPLE
- PREP/COOK TIME: 30 MIN
- ALL SEASONS

**FOR THE CURRY**

2 tablespoons **olive oil**
1 **onion**, chopped
2 **cloves garlic**, minced
1 **red pepper**, diced
1 **carrot**, sliced
1 (15½-ounce) can (400 grams) **chickpeas**, drained and rinsed
2 cups (400 milliliters) **coconut milk**
2 tablespoons **red curry paste**
1 tablespoon **peanut butter**
1 tablespoon **soy sauce**
1 tablespoon **nutritional yeast**

**TO SERVE**

cooked **rice** or **naan**
a few leaves **fresh cilantro** (optional)
a handful of **peanuts**, chopped
**salt** and **pepper**, to taste

**1.** In a large saucepan, heat the olive oil over medium heat. Add the chopped onion and sauté until soft and lightly browned.

**2.** Add the garlic and cook for another minute, stirring constantly to prevent burning.

**3.** Add the diced red pepper and the sliced carrot. Cook for a few minutes until vegetables begin to soften slightly.

**4.** Add drained chickpeas to the pan and mix well with the vegetables.

**5.** Pour coconut milk into the saucepan and add red curry paste, peanut butter, soy sauce, and nutritional yeast. Season with salt and pepper to taste. Mix ingredients well.

**6.** Let curry simmer over low heat for 15 to 20 minutes or until the vegetables are tender and the sauce has thickened.

**7.** Meanwhile, chop the peanuts using a large knife.

**8.** Serve with rice or naan, and sprinkle with fresh cilantro, if desired, and chopped peanuts.

FOR 100 G

| protein: **4.2 g** | carbohydrates: **10 g** | lipids: **13.4 g** |
|---|---|---|

PER PORTION (400 G)

| protein: **17 g** | carbohydrates: **40.2 g** | lipids: **53.5 g** |
|---|---|---|

- FOR 4 PEOPLE
- PREP/COOK TIME: 55 MIN
- ALL SEASONS

# SMASH SEITAN-BEAN BURGER

**FOR THE SEITAN "STEAK" WITH KIDNEY BEANS**

½ (15½-ounce) can (200 grams), **kidney beans**, drained and rinsed
2 tablespoons **soy sauce**
2 tablespoons **nutritional yeast**
1 tablespoon **tomato paste**
1 teaspoon **ground smoked paprika**
1 teaspoon **garlic powder**
1 teaspoon **onion powder**
½ teaspoon **black pepper**
½ teaspoon **salt**
1½ cups (200 grams) **vital wheat gluten flour**

**FOR THE BURGER**

½ **red onion**, peeled
large sweet-and-sour **pickles**
**iceberg lettuce**
1 large **tomato** (optional, depending on the season)
1 teaspoon **olive oil**
4 slices **plant-based "cheese"**
1 tablespoon **plant butter**, unsalted
4 **burger buns**
plant-based **barbecue sauce**

**1.** In a blender, combine kidney beans with soy sauce, nutritional yeast, tomato paste, ground smoked paprika, garlic powder, onion powder, black pepper, and salt. Blend until smooth.

**2.** In a large bowl, mix the red bean puree and the vital wheat gluten flour. Knead and mix well for about 5 minutes until the dough is elastic.

**3.** Divide the dough into 4 golf ball–sized portions. Place each dough ball between 2 sheets of baking paper and flatten to obtain 4 "steaks."

**4.** Place the 4 "steaks" in a steamer basket lined with perforated paper. Steam and cook covered for 10 to 15 minutes.

**5.** Meanwhile, finely slice the onion, cut the pickles into strips, roughly chop the salad, and cut 4 large slices of tomato.

**6.** Heat a pan with olive oil, place the "steaks" in it, and press firmly with a spatula to flatten (hence the name "smash burger"). Let cook, 3 to 4 minutes on each side.

**7.** Place a slice of plant-based "cheese" on each "steak" 1 minute before the end of cooking and cover with a lid allowing the "cheese" to melt.

**8.** Keep "steaks" warm, melt plant butter in the same pan, and grill the back of the buns.

**9.** Assemble your burger by spreading a tablespoon of barbecue sauce on the bun, add "steak," lettuce, tomato, pickles, and red onions. Finish with a little more barbecue sauce on top, and close.

FOR 100 G

| protein: **19.9 g** | carbohydrates: **24.1 g** | lipids: **4.2 g** |
|---|---|---|

PER PORTION (400 G)

| protein: **49.2 g** | carbohydrates: **59.9 g** | lipids: **10.4 g** |
|---|---|---|

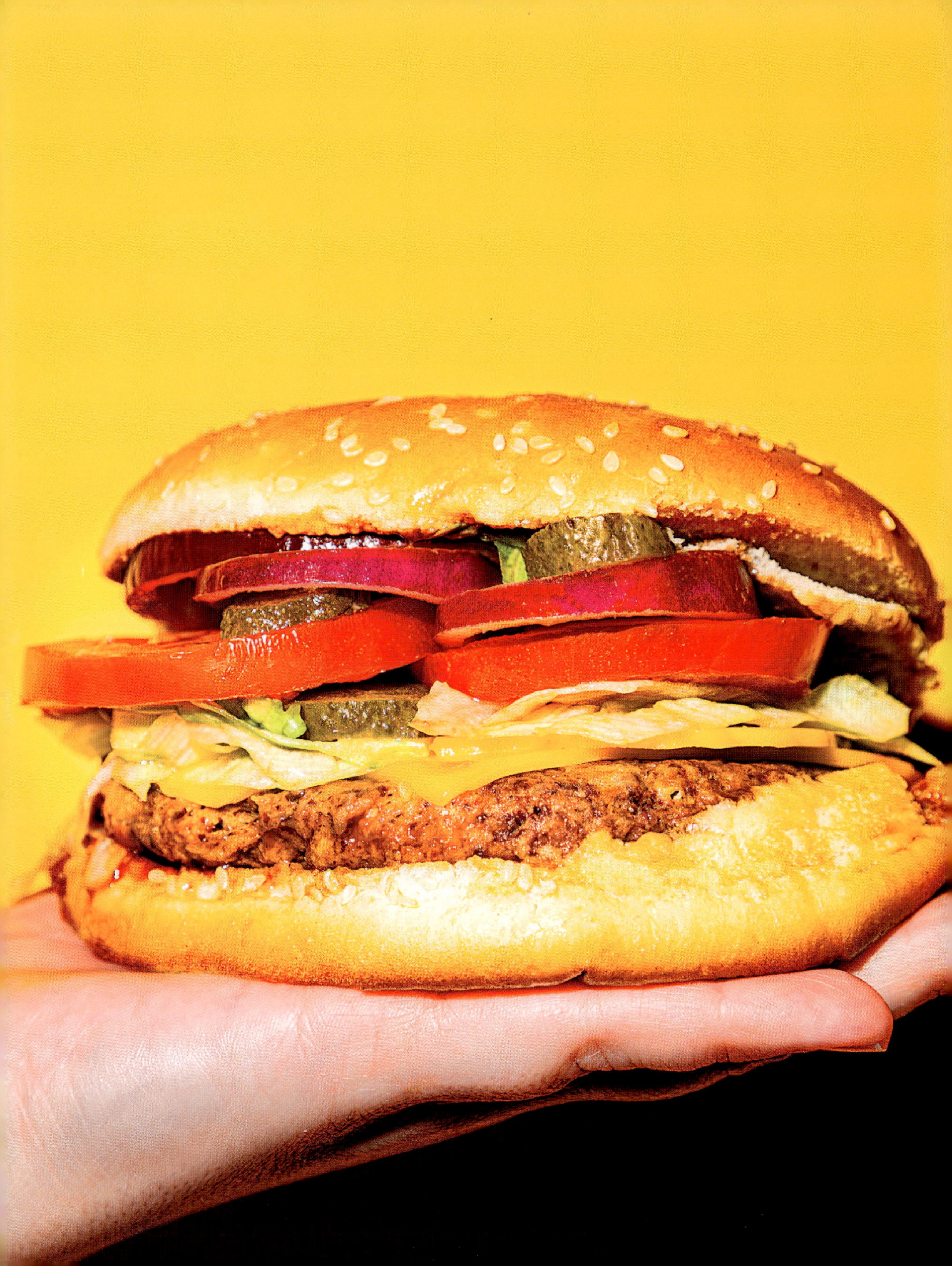

- FOR 3 PEOPLE
- PREP/COOK TIME: 25 MIN
- ALL SEASONS

# TAGLIATELLE WITH TOFU AND MUSHROOMS

14 ounces (400 grams) **tagliatelle pasta**
7 ounces (200 grams) **white mushrooms**
1 tablespoon **plant butter**, unsalted
1 tablespoon **garlic powder**
2 tablespoons **soy sauce**
10½ ounces (300 grams) **soft tofu**
2 tablespoons **truffle oil** (optional), divided
a few leaves **fresh parsley**, chopped
freshly **ground pepper**

**1.** Start by cooking your pasta according to the package instructions, until *al dente*. Reserve 1 cup of pasta water, drain the rest, and set aside.

**2.** Cut the mushrooms into slices. In a skillet over medium heat, melt the plant butter, and sauté mushrooms until tender. Add garlic powder and soy sauce to the pan. Mix well and let cook for a few more minutes to allow the flavors to develop.

**3.** Transfer about ¾ of the cooked mushrooms to a blender. Add soft tofu and most of the truffle oil, if desired, and blend until smooth and creamy.

**4.** Pour the creamy mixture into the pan with the remaining mushrooms. Stir and dilute with the reserved pasta water to thin the texture if necessary.

**5.** Add the cooked pasta to the pan with the mushroom sauce. Mix gently, so that it soaks up the sauce well.

**6.** Arrange the pasta on a plate, garnished with a little freshly ground pepper, chopped fresh parsley, and a drizzle of extra truffle oil, if desired.

## Tip

Truffles are sensitive to heat, so don't let them cook or simmer too much (it is better to add a drizzle after cooking). It is also optional in this recipe, and a good quality olive oil can completely do the trick.

FOR 100 G

| protein: **7.7 g** | carbohydrates: **26.2 g** | lipids: **7.5 g** |
|---|---|---|

PER SERVING (320 G)

| protein: **24.6 g** | carbohydrates: **83.8 g** | lipids: **23.7 g** |
|---|---|---|

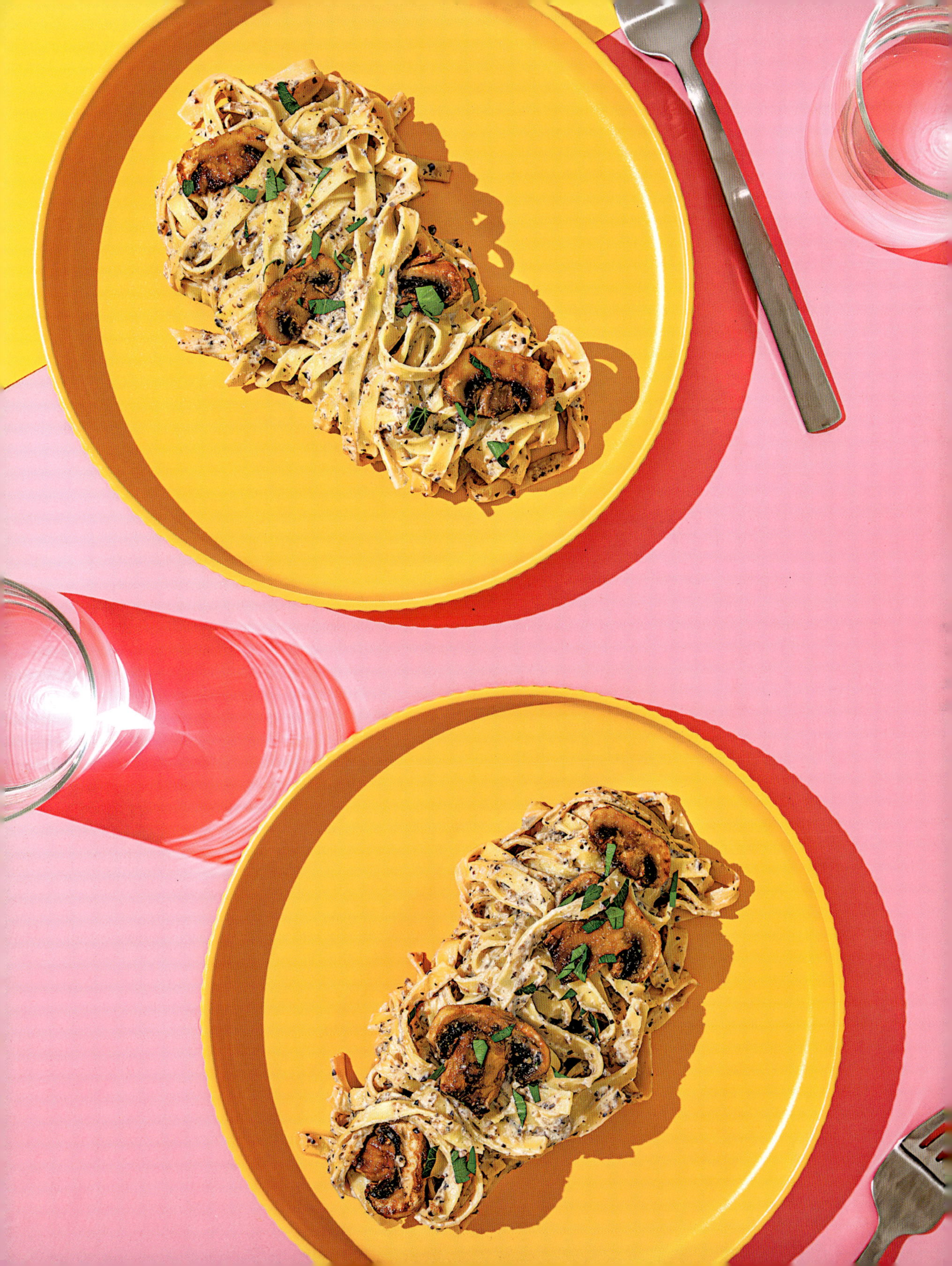

- FOR 4 PEOPLE
- PREP/COOK TIME: 55 MIN
- ALL SEASONS

# STUFFED SWEET POTATOES WITH TEMPEH

2 **sweet potatoes**
2 tablespoons **olive oil**
1 **onion**, chopped
2 **cloves garlic**, chopped
10½ ounces (300 grams) **tempeh**
2 tablespoons **soy sauce**
3½ ounces (100 grams) **mushrooms**, sliced
⅓ (15¼-ounce) can (150 grams) **corn**, drained and rinsed
3½ ounces (100 grams) **fresh spinach**, chopped
**plant-based grated "cheese"** to garnish (optional)
**salt** and **pepper**, to taste

**1.** Preheat the oven to 350°F.

**2.** Wash the sweet potatoes, then pierce them several times with a fork. Wrap in tinfoil, and place on a baking sheet. Bake for 35 to 45 minutes, or until tender.

**3.** Meanwhile, in a skillet, heat 1 tablespoons of olive oil over medium heat. Add the chopped onion and garlic and brown them until golden brown. Cut the block of tempeh into strips and add them to the pan. Cook until golden and crispy. Deglaze with soy sauce. Add the sliced mushrooms and corn to the pan and sauté the vegetables until the mushrooms have released all water. Add the chopped spinach to the pan and cook until wilted. Season with salt and pepper to taste. Mix well.

**4.** Once the sweet potatoes are cooked, remove them from the oven and let them cool slightly, without turning off the oven. Cut them in half lengthwise.

**5.** Using a spoon, carefully scoop out the flesh of the cooked sweet potatoes, leaving a thin layer of flesh inside the skin. Mix the flesh in the pan with the other ingredients. Fill the hollowed-out sweet potato halves with the tempeh, spinach, mushroom, and corn mixture. Sprinkle with the plant-based grated "cheese" and drizzle with 1 tablespoon of olive oil.

**6.** Put the stuffed sweet potatoes back in the oven for about 10 minutes. Serve immediately!

FOR 100 G

| protein: **6.5 g** | carbohydrates: **13.2 g** | lipids: **5.7 g** |
|---|---|---|

PER PORTION (300 G)

| protein: **19.5 g** | carbohydrates: **39.7 g** | lipids: **17 g** |
|---|---|---|

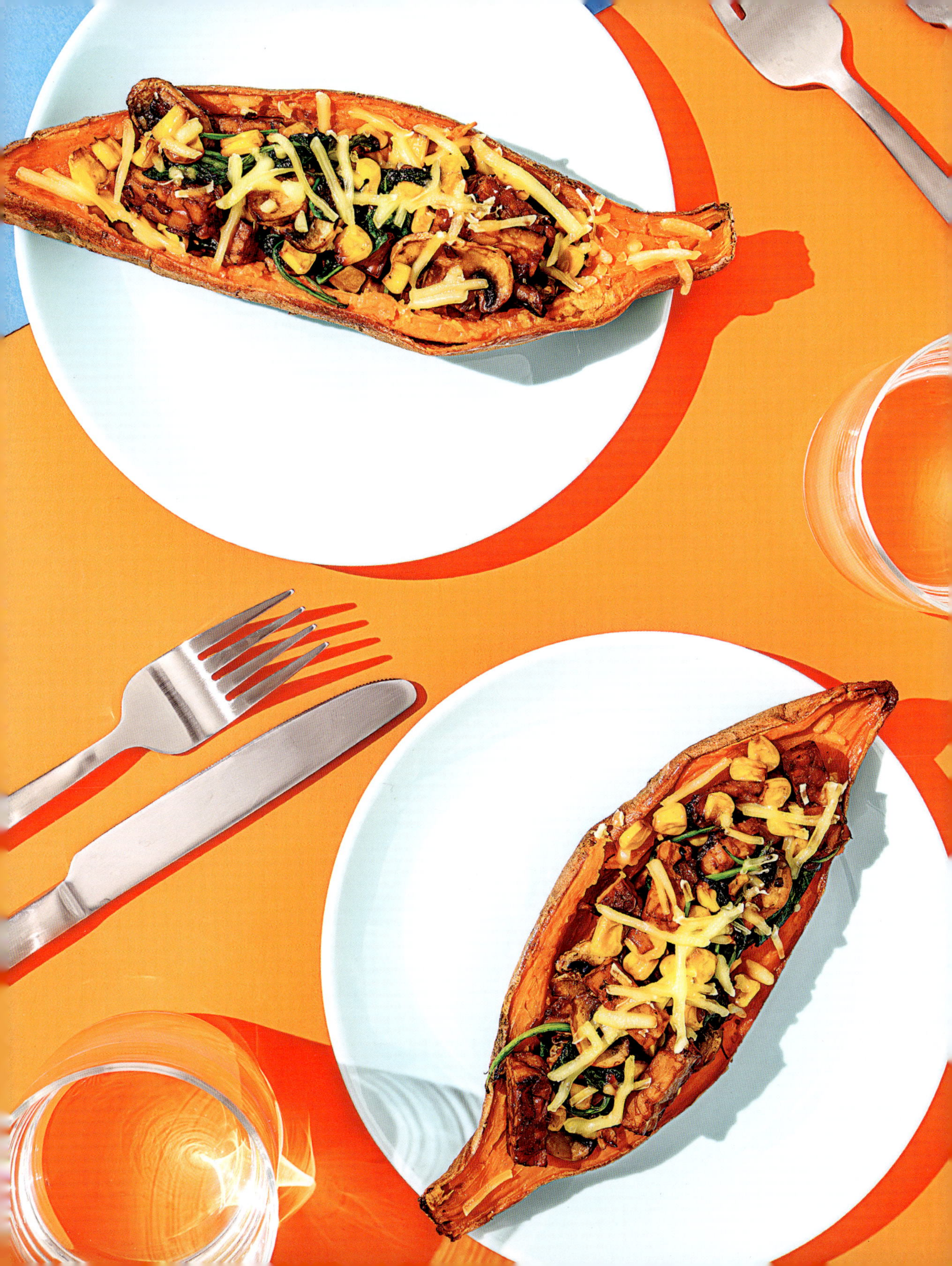

- FOR 4 PEOPLE
- PREP/COOK TIME: 1 HOUR
- REST TIME: 5 MIN
- ALL SEASONS

# CHILI SIN CARNE WITH QUINOA AND SWEET POTATO

1 cup (200 grams) **quinoa**

**FOR THE CHILI**

2 **sweet potatoes**
1 **red pepper**
1 **onion**
2 **cloves garlic**
2 tablespoons **olive oil**
2 teaspoons **ground smoked paprika**
1 teaspoon **ground cumin**
½ (15½-ounce) can (200 grams) kidney **beans**, drained and rinsed
1 (15-ounce) can (400 grams) **crushed tomatoes**
**salt** and **pepper**, to taste

**TO SERVE**

a few leaves **fresh cilantro**
½ **lime,** cut into wedges
1 **jalapeño**, sliced

**1.** Rinse the quinoa in cold water. In a saucepan, boil about 2 cups of water. Add the quinoa, reduce the heat, and simmer for 15 minutes, or until cooked and water is absorbed. Remove from the heat and let stand covered for 5 minutes. Fluff the quinoa with a fork and set aside.

**2.** Prepare your ingredients: peel and cut the sweet potatoes into cubes, seed and cut the red pepper into thin strips, chop the onion, and mince the garlic.

**3.** In a large skillet, heat the olive oil over medium heat. Add the onion, garlic, and spices and sauté for 2 to 3 minutes until golden and fragrant.

**4.** Add the sweet potatoes and the red pepper to pan. Sauté for about 5 minutes until the vegetables begin to soften.

**5.** Add the drained kidney beans and crushed tomatoes. Season with salt and pepper to taste. Simmer for about 10 to 15 minutes until the sweet potatoes are tender.

**6.** Serve the quinoa hot in a deep plate and pour a generous amount of chili on top.

**7.** Serve hot, garnished with fresh cilantro, lime wedges, and jalapeño slices.

FOR 100 G

| protein: **4.7 g** | carbohydrates: **21.4 g** | lipids: **3.7 g** |
|---|---|---|

PER PORTION (350 G)

| protein: **16.5 g** | carbohydrates: **74.9 g** | lipids: **12.9 g** |
|---|---|---|

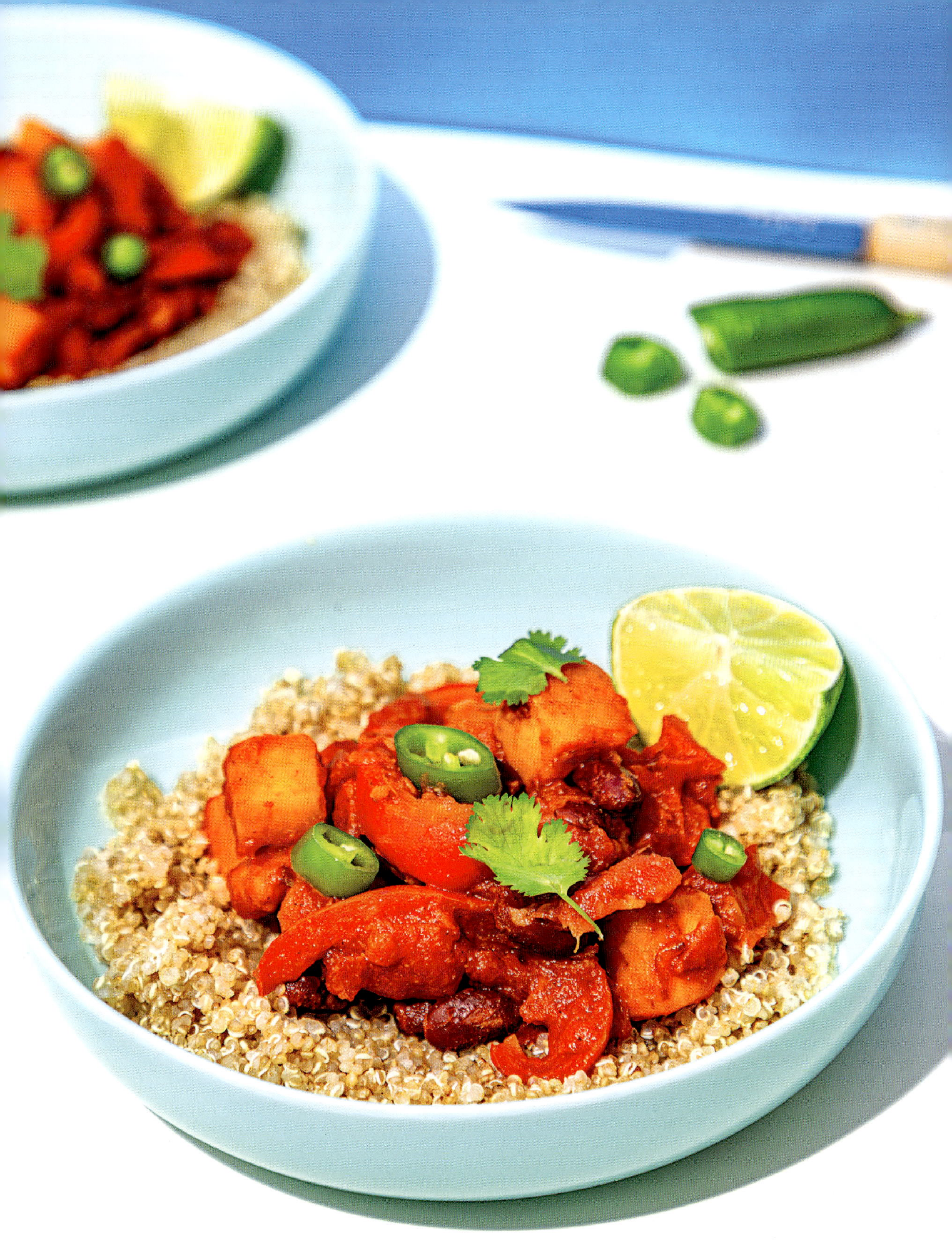

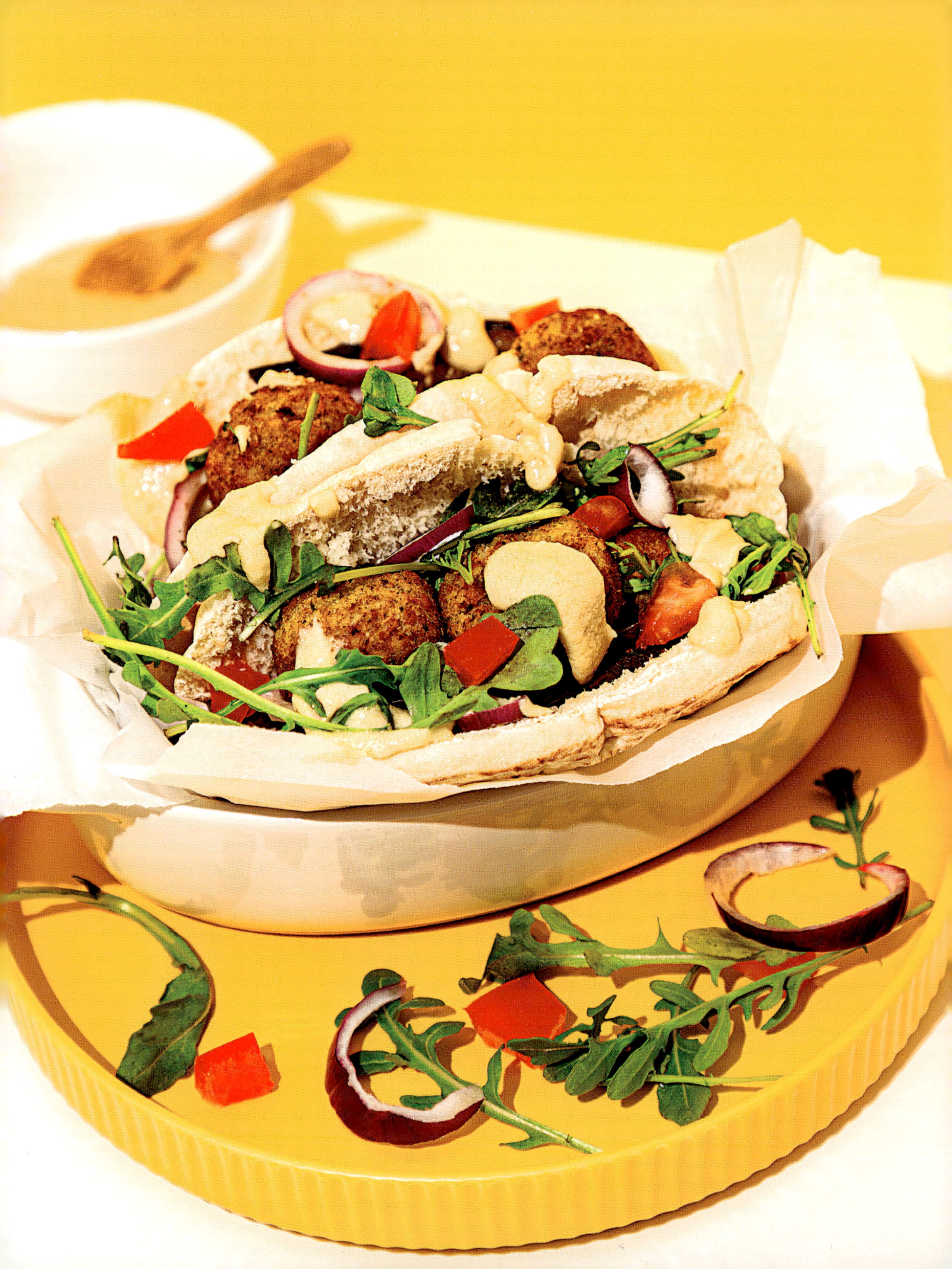

# PITA BREAD WITH FALAFELS AND TAHINI SAUCE

- FOR 4 PEOPLE
- PREP/COOK TIME: 35 MIN
- SUMMER

**FOR THE PITA BREAD AND FILLING**

1 **eggplant**
a drizzle of **olive oil**
2 teaspoons **ground smoked paprika**
1 teaspoon **garlic powder**
**salt** and **pepper**, to taste
10 **falafel**
1 **tomato**
1 **red onion**
4 pieces **pita bread**
¼ cup **pumpkin seed "cream cheese"** (see page 28, Pumpkin Seed and Chickpea "Skyr")
a few handfuls of **arugula**

**FOR THE TAHINI VINAIGRETTE SAUCE**

2 tablespoons **tahini**
1 tablespoon **olive oil**
1 teaspoons **maple syrup**
**juice of ½ lemon**
1 tablespoon **water**
**salt** and **pepper**, to taste

**1.** Start by preheating the oven to 400°F.

**2.** Cut the eggplant into slices about ½ inch thick. Place the slices on a baking sheet covered with baking paper. Drizzle with olive oil, then season with ground smoked paprika, garlic powder, salt, and pepper. Bake for 20 to 25 minutes, or until tender and golden.

**3.** Meanwhile, prepare the falafel according to the package instructions.

**4.** Make the tahini vinaigrette by mixing all the ingredients in a bowl until smooth and creamy. Add a little more water if necessary to obtain desired consistency.

**5.** Cut the tomato into small cubes and cut the red onion into thin slices.

**6.** Once the eggplant slices are cooked, warm the pita bread in oven for a few minutes.

**7.** Assemble the pitas: Spread each pita with pumpkin seed cream cheese, add a few falafel, roasted eggplant slices, red onion slices, diced tomatoes, a handful of arugula, and drizzle generously with tahini vinaigrette. Fold the pitas and serve immediately.

## Tip

You can buy ready-to-eat plant-based "cream cheese" or make it at home by following the Pumpkin Seed and Chickpea "Skyr" recipe (see page 28).

FOR 100 G

| protein: **5.6 g** | carbohydrates: **20.9 g** | lipids: **4.9 g** |
|---|---|---|

PER PORTION (300 G)

| protein: **16.7 g** | carbohydrates: **62.7 g** | lipids: **14.6 g** |
|---|---|---|

- FOR 2 PEOPLE
- PREP TIME: 35 MIN
- ALL SEASONS

# COCONUT DAHL WITH LENTILS AND TOFU

½ cup (100 grams) **red lentils**
7 ounces (200 grams) **firm tofu**
2 tablespoons **olive oil**, divided
2 tablespoons **soy sauce**
1 **onion**, chopped
1 **clove garlic**, minced
1 **carrot**, cut into slices
2 teaspoons **curry powder**
¾ cup (150 milliliters) **coconut cream**
⅔ (15-ounce) can (300 milliliters) **crushed tomatoes**
½ cup (100 milliliters) **vegetable broth** (optional)
some leaves of **fresh cilantro**
freshly **ground pepper**

**1.** Rinse the lentils in clean water and drain.

**2.** Cut the tofu into small cubes and brown it in a pan with 1 tablespoon of olive oil until golden brown. Deglaze with soy sauce, then set aside.

**3.** In the same pan, with the remaining olive oil, sauté the chopped onion until translucent. Then add the minced garlic and sliced carrot. Add curry powder, drained lentils, coconut cream, and crushed tomatoes. Mix well and reduce to low heat. Let simmer, stirring regularly. You can add a little vegetable stock if necessary. When cooked, add previously prepared tofu and mix well.

**4.** When ready to serve, garnish with remaining coconut cream, chopped fresh cilantro, and freshly ground pepper.

## Tip

The soy sauce will already have salted the dish, but you can add a little salt according to your taste. You can serve this dish with a side of rice.

FOR 100 G

| protein: **6.3 g** | carbohydrates: **9.9 g** | lipids: **6.4 g** |
|---|---|---|

PER PORTION (350 G)

| protein: **22 g** | carbohydrates: **34.6 g** | lipids: **22.3 g** |
|---|---|---|

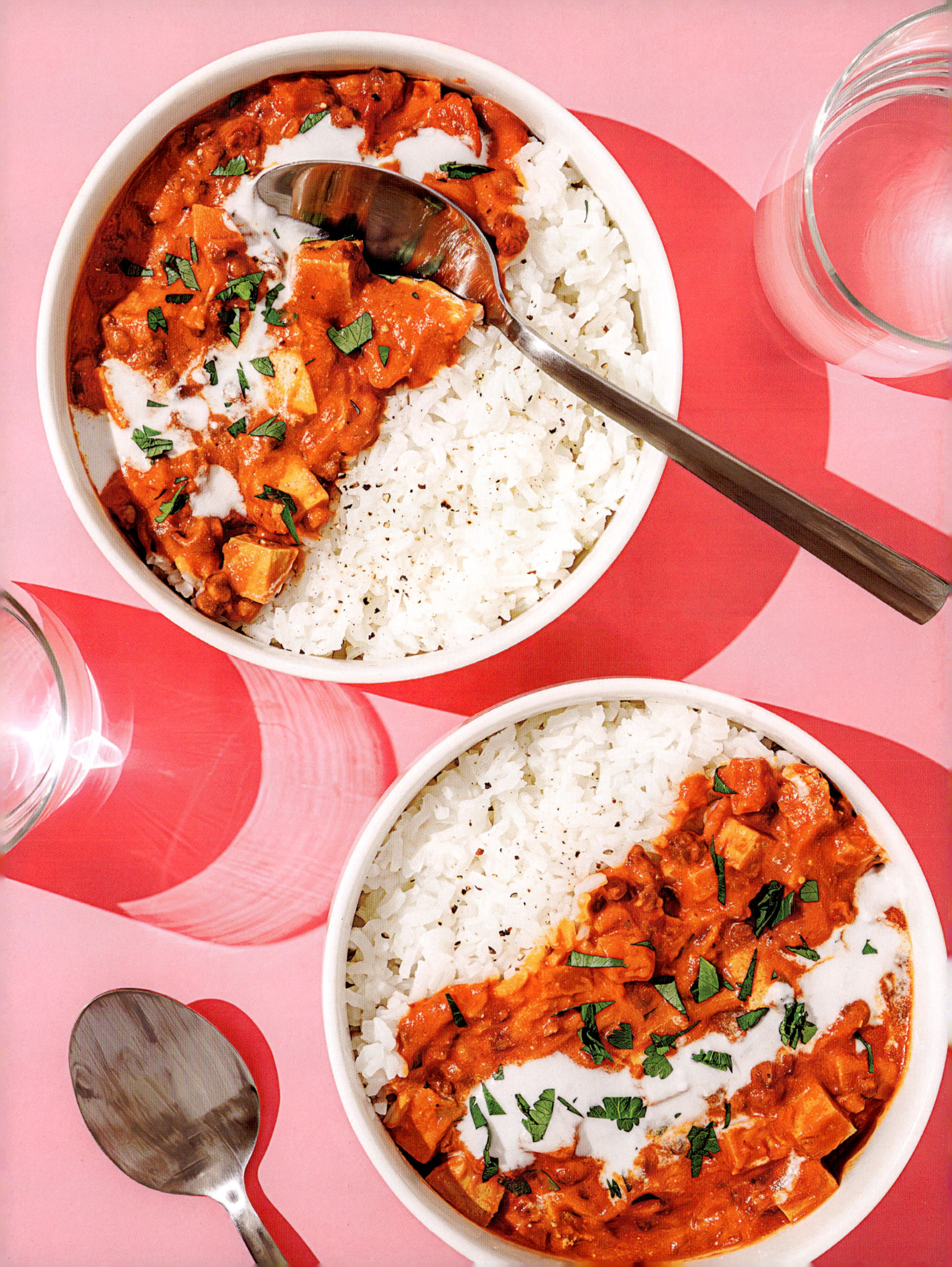

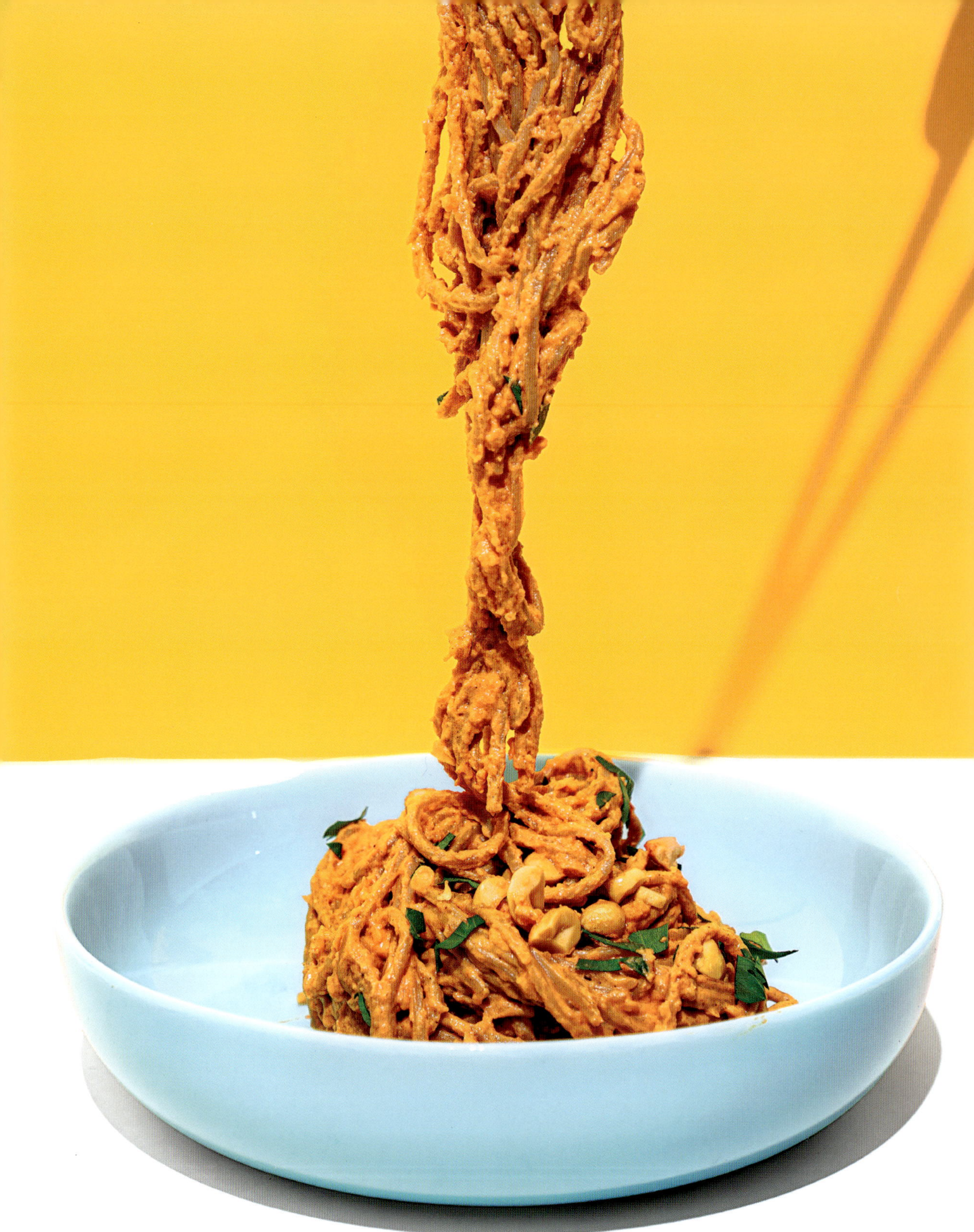

# SOBA NOODLES WITH PEANUT SAUCE

- FOR 2 PEOPLE
- PREP/COOK TIME: 25 MIN
- ALL SEASONS

½ pound (250 grams) **soba noodles**

**FOR THE PEANUT SAUCE**
a drizzle of **olive oil**
1 **onion**, finely chopped
1 **clove garlic**, minced
1 teaspoon **ground smoked paprika**
⅓ cup (50 grams) **peanuts**, whole
10½ ounces (300 grams) **soft tofu**
2 tablespoons **nutritional yeast**
1 tablespoon **tomato paste**
**juice of ½ lemon**
**red chili pepper**, to taste

**TO SERVE**
a few leaves of **fresh cilantro**, chopped
2 handfuls of **peanuts**, chopped

**1.** In a saucepan, brown the finely chopped onion, minced garlic, and ground smoked paprika in a pan with a drizzle of olive oil until lightly browned and fragrant. Transfer the mixture to a blender with all other sauce ingredients, and blend until smooth and consistent.

**2.** In the same pan, cook the blended sauce over low heat for a few minutes, stirring regularly, to warm it up and let the flavors develop.

**3.** Meanwhile, cook the soba noodles according to the package instructions. Once cooked, set aside ½ cup of pasta water, drain the rest, and set noodles aside.

**4.** Dip the cooked noodles into hot sauce and mix gently to coat evenly. Use the reserved pasta water to thin if the sauce is too thick.

**5.** Arrange the noodles in deep plates and sprinkle with finely chopped fresh cilantro and chopped peanuts.

## Tip

Eat with chopsticks.

FOR 100 G

| protein: **8.4 g** | carbohydrates: **26 g** | lipids: **6.4 g** |
|---|---|---|

PER PORTION (350 G)

| protein: **29.4 g** | carbohydrates: **91.2 g** | lipids: **22.6 g** |
|---|---|---|

- FOR 4 PEOPLE
- PREP/COOK TIME: 40 MIN
- ALL SEASONS

# TOFU-STUFFED CABBAGE LEAVES

**FOR THE STUFFED CABBAGE LEAVES**

8 **green cabbage** leaves
1 tablespoon **olive oil**
7 ounces (200 grams) **mushrooms**, finely chopped
7 ounces (200 grams) **firm tofu**, crumbled
1 **carrot**, grated
1 **onion**, chopped
2 tablespoons **soy sauce**
**salt** and **pepper**, to taste

**FOR THE "YOGURT" SAUCE**

7 ounces (200 grams) **plant-based "yogurt"**
a few stems **fresh dill**, chopped
a few stems **fresh chives**, chopped
1 tablespoon **olive oil**
1 tablespoons fresh **lemon juice**
**salt** and **pepper**, to taste

**1.** Bring a large pot of salted water to a boil. Dip the cabbage leaves in boiling water for about 5 minutes, or until tender. You can plunge cabbage leaves into cold water to stop the cooking. Drain and set aside.

**2.** In a skillet, heat olive oil over medium heat. Add the finely chopped mushrooms, crumbled tofu, grated carrot, and chopped onion. Sauté everything for 5 to 7 minutes until the vegetables are tender.

**3.** Stir the soy sauce into the mushroom and tofu mixture. Season with salt and pepper to taste. Let cook for a few more minutes to let the flavors blend.

**4.** Preheat the oven to 350°F.

**5.** On a work surface, spread out a cabbage leaf and place a portion of the mushroom and tofu mixture in the center. Roll the cabbage leaf around the filling. Repeat with the remaining cabbage leaves and filling.

**6.** In a baking dish, arrange the stuffed cabbage leaves. Cook for 10 to 15 minutes, or until they are lightly browned.

**7.** Meanwhile, prepare the sauce by mixing all the ingredients.

**8.** When ready to serve, divide the sauce between 4 soup plates and place the stuffed cabbage leaves on top.

FOR 100 G

| protein: **5.6 g** | carbohydrates: **5.7 g** | lipids: **6.5 g** |
|---|---|---|

PER PORTION (350 G)

| protein: **19.6 g** | carbohydrates: **19.9 g** | lipids: **22.7 g** |
|---|---|---|

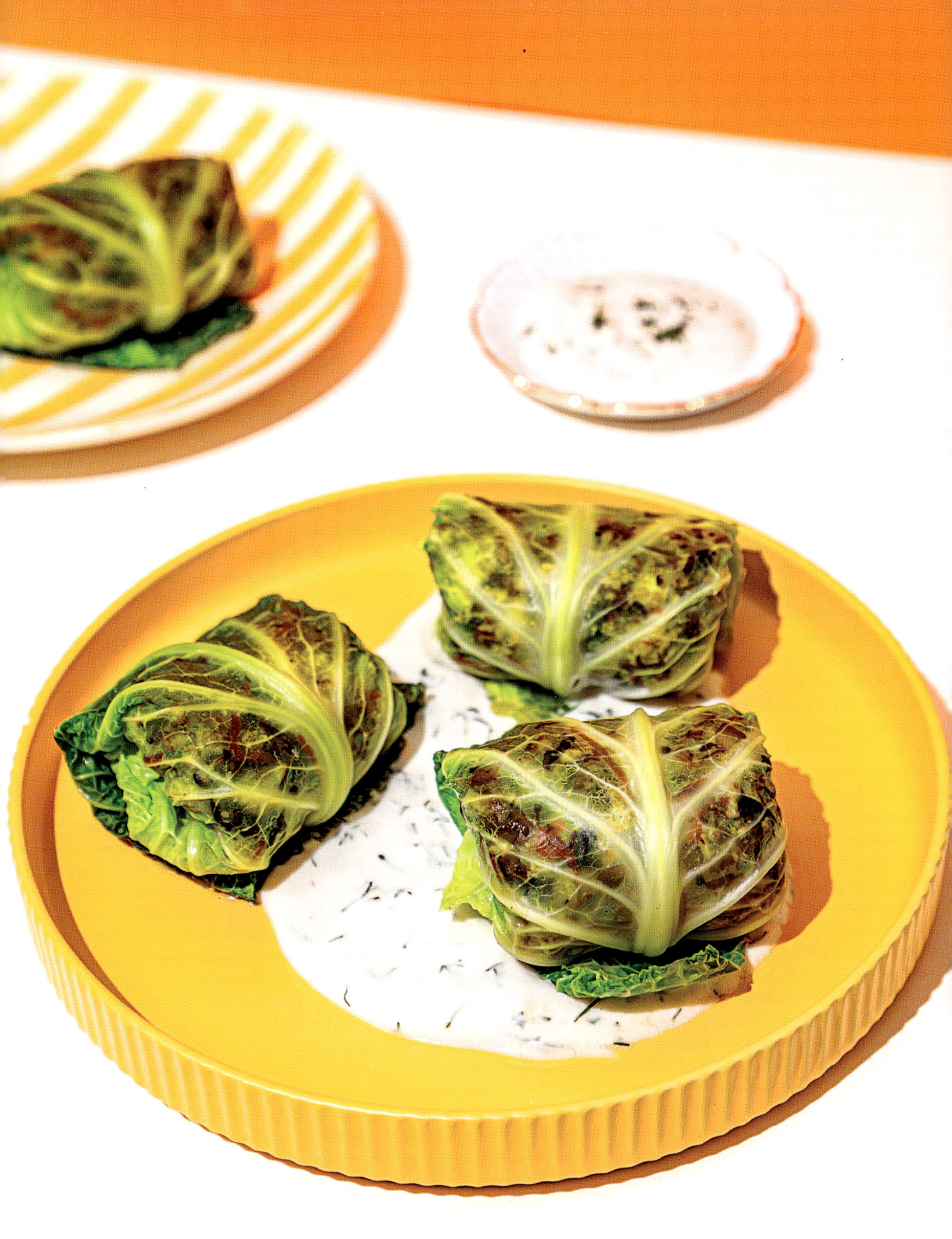

- FOR 2 PEOPLE
- PREP/COOK TIME: 35 MIN
- SUMMER WITHOUT BROCCOLI, OR FALL

# FRIED BROCCOLI AND QUINOA CAKES

½ cup (90 grams) **quinoa**
1 **onion**
1½ cups (140 grams) **broccoli**
2 tablespoons **nutritional yeast**
2 tablespoons **chickpea flour**
2 tablespoons **olive oil**
1 teaspoon **salt**
½ teaspoon **pepper**

**1.** Cook the quinoa according to the package instructions. Let it cool once cooked.

**2.** Meanwhile, finely chop the onion and cut the broccoli into florets. Cook the broccoli florets for 10 minutes in boiling water, then mash them into a puree.

**3.** In a large bowl, mix the cooked quinoa, broccoli puree, chopped onion, nutritional yeast, chickpea flour, salt, and pepper. Make sure all ingredients are mixed well.

**4.** Heat a skillet with some olive oil over medium heat. Take a portion of the quinoa and broccoli mixture to form a small, thick patty. Place in hot skillet.

**5.** Repeat the process with the remaining mixture, being careful not to crowd the pan.

**6.** Pan-fry the cakes for 4 to 5 minutes on each side, or until golden and crispy.

## Tip

You can serve the cakes with soy sauce or prepare a tahini sauce (see page 24, Salty Buckwheat Waffles with Tahini Sauce).

FOR 100 G

| protein: **6.8 g** | carbohydrates: **21.9 g** | lipids: **8.3 g** |
|---|---|---|

PER PORTION (180 G)

| protein: **12.2 g** | carbohydrates: **39.4 g** | lipids: **14.9 g** |
|---|---|---|

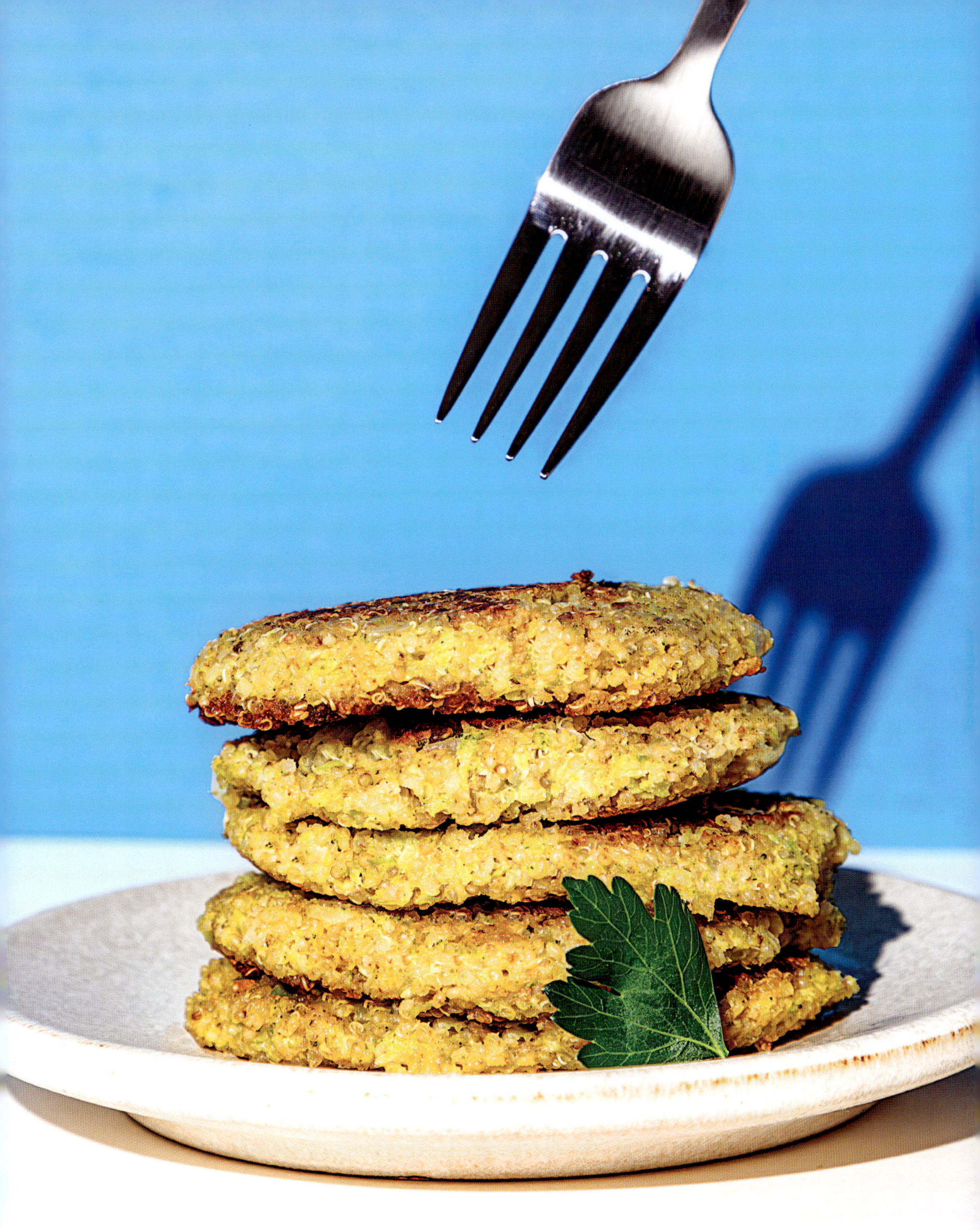

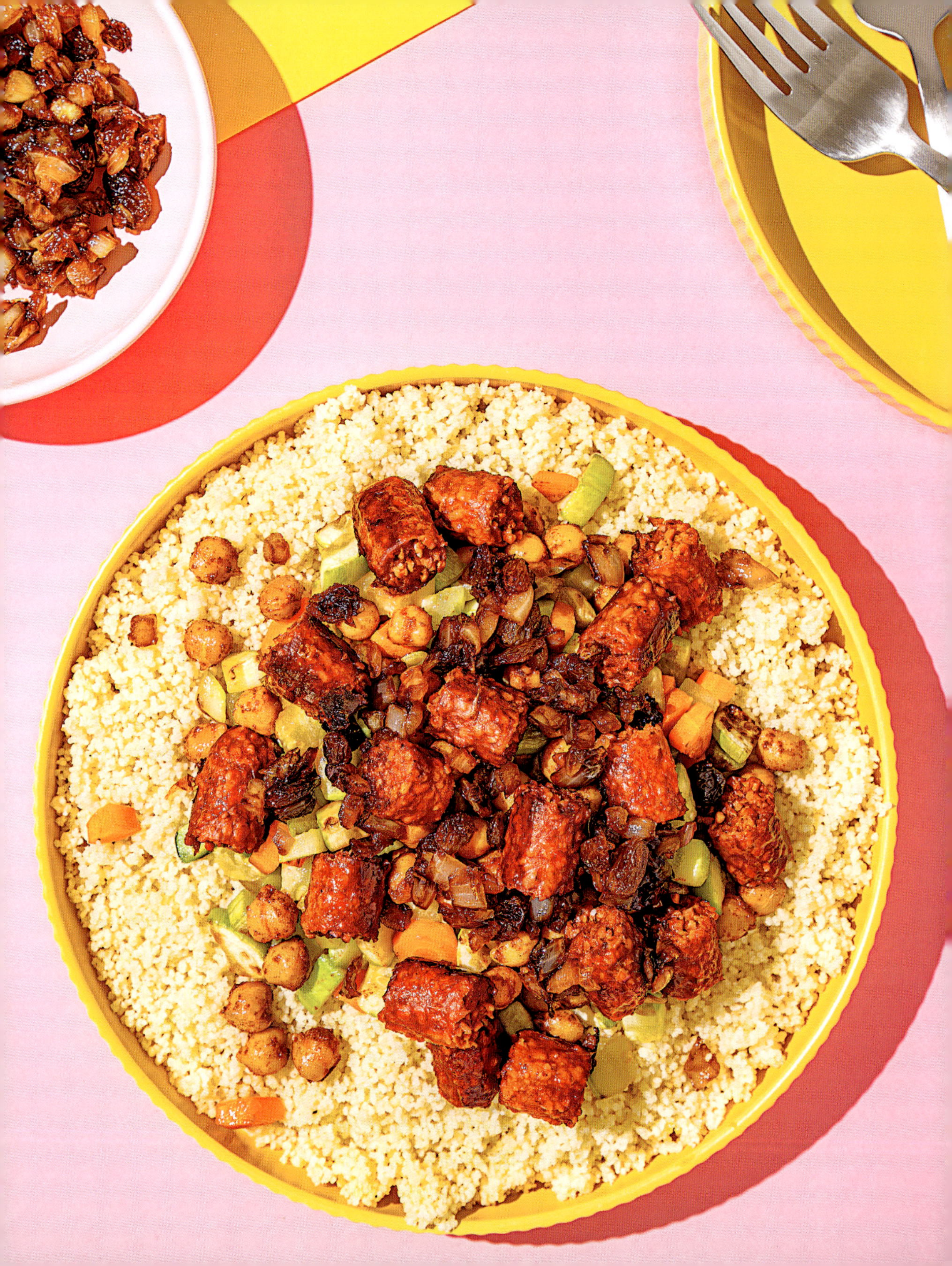

# SPICY COUSCOUS BOWL WITH CHICKPEAS AND "*MERGUEZ*"

- FOR 4 PEOPLE
- PREP/COOK TIME: 25 MIN
- ALL SEASONS

**FOR THE COUSCOUS**

7 ounces (200 grams) **couscous**
1 **carrot**
1 **zucchini**
1 tablespoon **olive oil**
¼ (15½-ounce) can (100 grams) **chickpeas**, drained and rinsed
1 teaspoon **cumin**
1 teaspoon **ground smoked paprika**
4 **plant-based "*merguez* sausages"**
salt and **pepper**, to taste

**FOR THE *TFAYA***

4 **onions**
2 tablespoons **olive oil**
2 tablespoons **sugar**
2 teaspoons **ground cinnamon**
1 teaspoon **ground ginger**
¼ cup (50 grams) **raisins**

**TO SERVE**

2 teaspoons **harissa** (optional)

**1.** Prepare the couscous according to the instructions on the package.

**2.** While the couscous is cooking, prepare the *tfaya*. Start by finely chopping the onions and brown them over medium heat in a saucepan with olive oil. When starting to be translucent, add the sugar, spices, and raisins, and let everything stew, stirring regularly.

**3.** Meanwhile, prepare your vegetables by peeling and dicing the carrot and zucchini, which you will brown in a hot pan with olive oil until soft. Then keep warm.

**4.** In the same pan, brown the chickpeas with cumin and ground smoked paprika. Keep warm.

**5.** Cut the plant-based "*merguez*" into slices and brown them in the pan according to the instructions on the packet.

**6.** The *tfaya* should have reduced. If it has a dark yellow color tending towards brown, it is ready! Then assemble the bowl: Place the semolina in deep plates and the *tfaya* on top.

**7.** Serve these plates with a little harissa on the side, if desired.

FOR 100 G

| protein: **4.2 g** | carbohydrates: **23.1 g** | lipids: **4.8 g** |
|---|---|---|

PER PORTION (350 G)

| protein: **14.7 g** | carbohydrates: **80.9 g** | lipids: **16.8 g** |
|---|---|---|

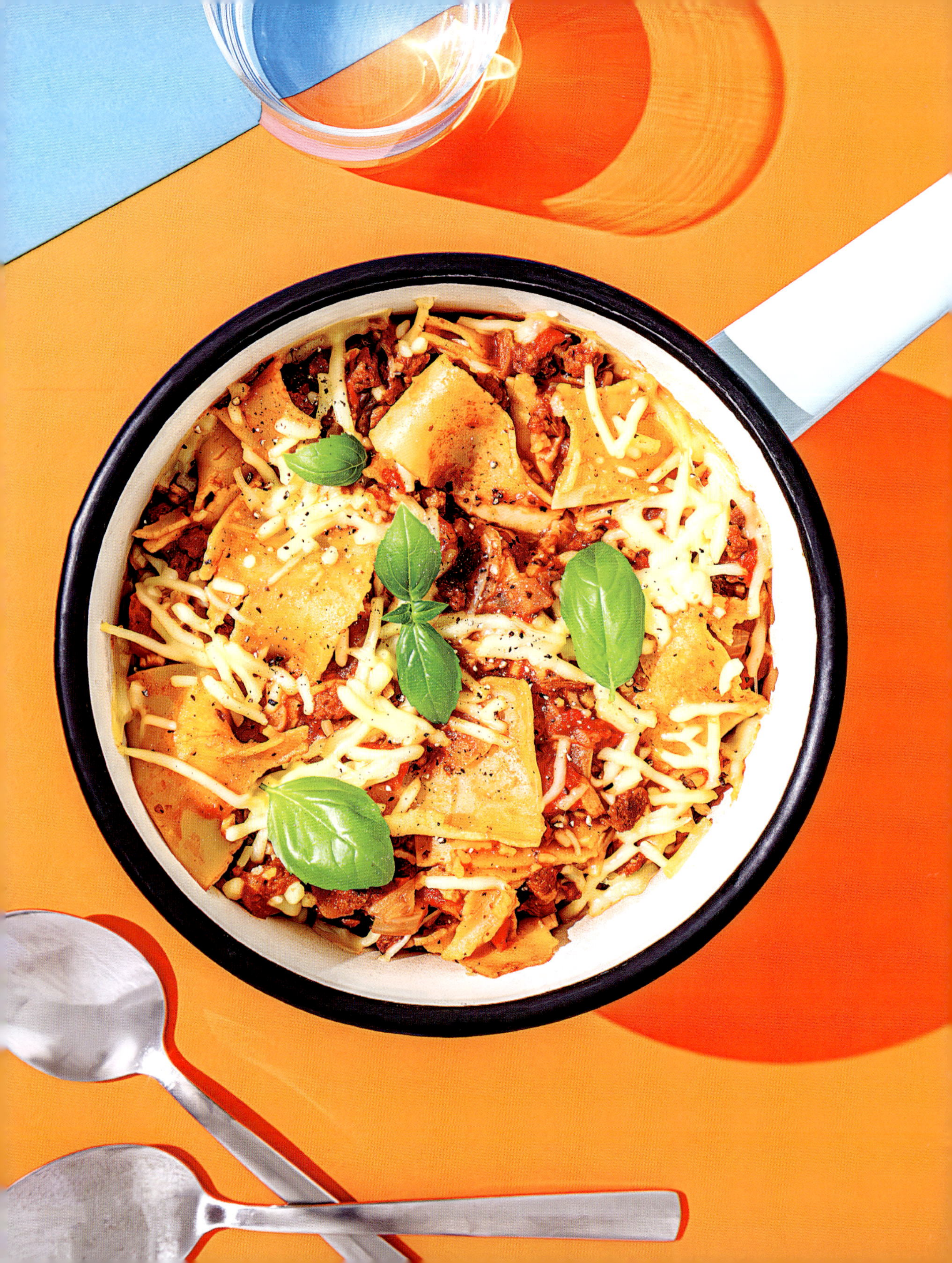

# ONE-POT LASAGNA

- FOR 3 PEOPLE
- PREP/COOK TIME: 40 MIN
- REST TIME: 5 MIN
- ALL SEASONS

2 tablespoons **olive oil**
1 **onion**, chopped
2 **cloves garlic**, minced
½ pound (250 grams) **plant-based ground "beef"**
1 (15-ounce) can (400 grams) **crushed tomatoes**
2 tablespoons **tomato paste**
2½ cups **vegetable broth**
1 teaspoon **dried oregano**
1 teaspoon **dried basil**
**salt** and freshly **ground pepper**, to taste
7 ounces (200 grams) **lasagna plates** (egg free)
1 cup (100 grams) **plant-based grated "cheese"** (optional)

**1.** In a large saucepan, heat the olive oil over medium heat. Add the chopped onion and minced garlic and sauté until golden and fragrant.

**2.** Add the plant-based ground "beef" to the pan and sauté until browned.

**3.** Stir in the crushed tomatoes, tomato paste, vegetable broth, dried oregano and dried basil, salt, and freshly ground pepper. Mix well.

**4.** Bring the mixture to a boil, then reduce the heat and simmer for about 10 minutes, stirring occasionally.

**5.** Add the lasagna plates to the pan. You can break them into 2 or 4 pieces if you prefer. Make sure they are well immersed in liquid. If necessary, add a little more broth. Cover the pan and simmer for about 15 minutes, or until pasta is cooked and sauce has thickened.

**6.** If desired, sprinkle some plant-based grated "cheese" on top. Cover the pan again and let it sit for a few minutes for the "cheese" to melt.

**7.** Once the "cheese" has melted, remove the pan from the heat. Add a little more freshly ground pepper, if desired, then serve hot.

## Tip

Instead of store-bought plant-based ground "beef," you can also make homemade Soy Bolognese (see page 64, Cauliflower Pizza with Soy Bolognese), or use lentils.

FOR 100 G

| protein: **6.7 g** | carbohydrates: **16.2 g** | lipids: **3.9 g** |
|---|---|---|

PER PORTION (350 G)

| protein: **23.3 g** | carbohydrates: **56.7 g** | lipids: **13.9 g** |
|---|---|---|

- FOR 4 PEOPLE
- PREP/COOK TIME: 35 MIN
- ALL SEASONS

# CORAL LENTIL SOUP WITH TEMPEH AND COCONUT

1 cup (200 grams) **red lentils**
1 **onion**, chopped
2 **cloves garlic**, minced
1 tablespoon **olive oil**
2 teaspoons **curry powder**
1 teaspoon **ground cumin** (optional)
1 teaspoon **ground coriander**
3½ ounces (100 grams) **tempeh**
1 **carrot**
2 tablespoons **soy sauce**
2½ cups (500 milliliters) **vegetable stock**
1 cup (200 milliliters) **coconut cream**
**fresh cilantro** leaves, to garnish (optional)

**1.** Rinse the red lentils, drain, then set aside.

**2.** In a saucepan, sauté the onion and garlic in olive oil until tender. Add all spices after 2 minutes of cooking.

**3.** Crumble the tempeh with your fingers and add to the pan. Then dice and add the carrot.

**4.** Mix over medium heat for 5 to 7 minutes, so that the mixture absorbs spices well and begins to brown lightly. Then deglaze with soy sauce before adding the lentils and vegetable stock to the pan.

**5.** Cook the lentils for about 15 minutes.

**6.** At the end of cooking, add the coconut cream. Mix well. Adjust the texture with an immersion blender, if you wish, and serve with a little fresh cilantro leaves.

FOR 100 G

| protein: **4 g** | carbohydrates: **8.5 g** | lipids: **5.6 g** |
|---|---|---|

PER PORTION (350 G)

| protein: **14 g** | carbohydrates: **29.8 g** | lipids: **19.6 g** |
|---|---|---|

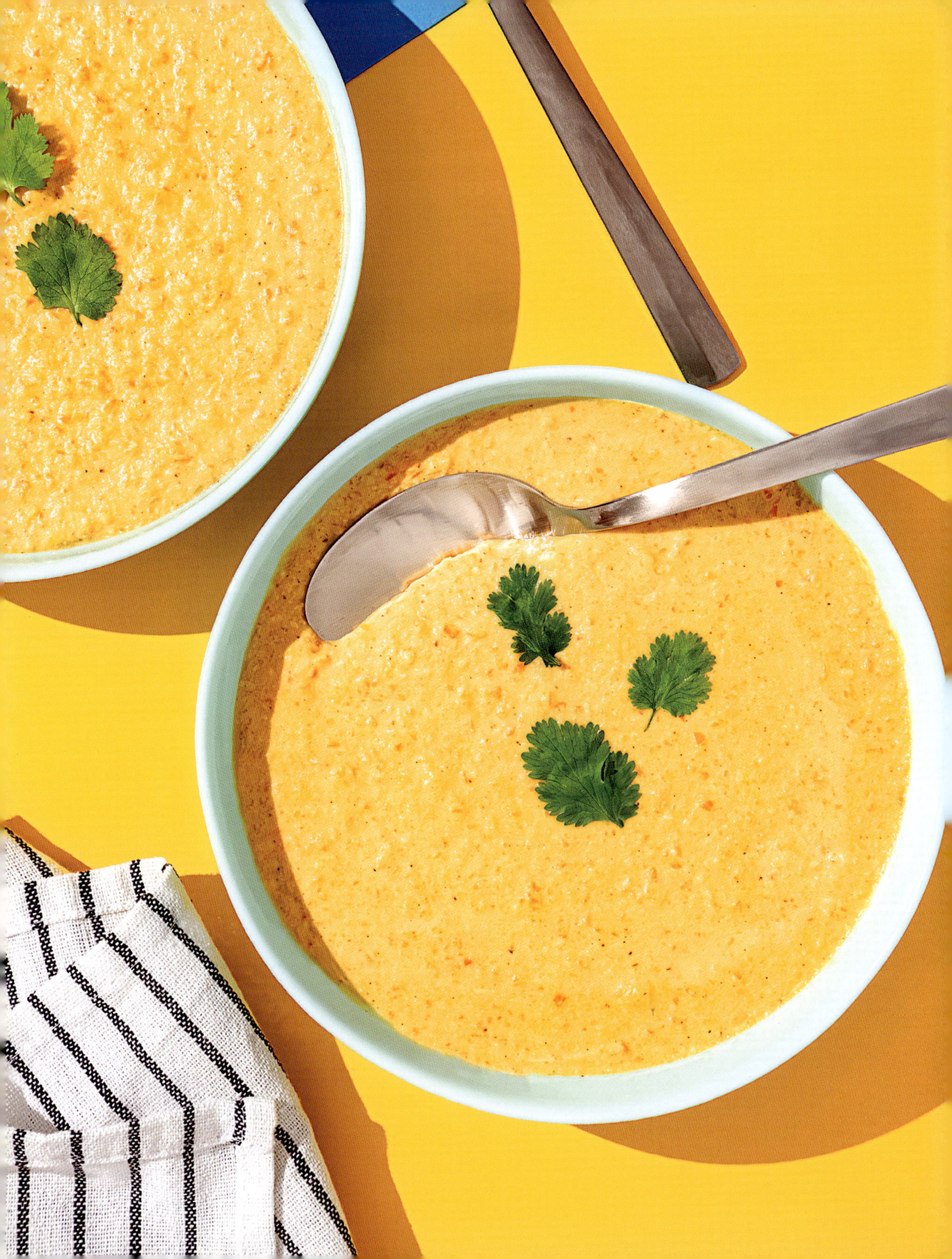

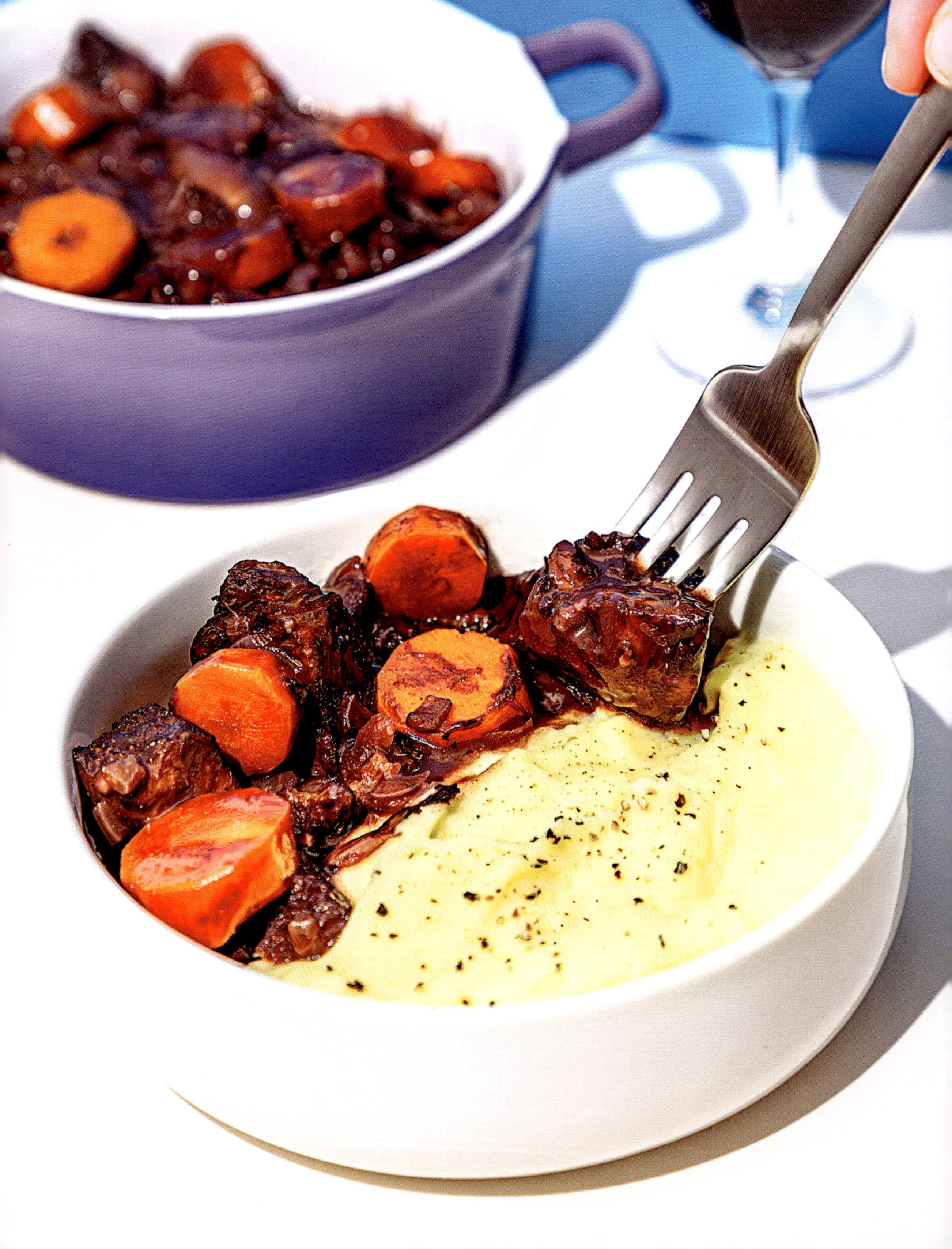

# BURGUNDY SEITAN STEW

- FOR 4 PEOPLE
- PREP/COOK TIME: 1 HOUR
- ALL SEASONS

2 teaspoons **plant butter**, unsalted
2 large **onions**, chopped
2 tablespoons **olive oil**
4 **carrots**, sliced
½ pound (250 grams) **white mushrooms**, quartered
1 pound (500 grams) **seitan** (store-bought or homemade seitan, see page 83, Caesar Salad with Homemade Seitan).
3 tablespoons **whole wheat flour**
approximately 2½ cups (500 milliliters) **red wine**
some sprigs **fresh thyme**
2 **bay leaves**
**salt** and **pepper**, to taste

**1.** In a large pot, melt the plant butter over medium heat.

**2.** Add the onions and sauté until soft and lightly browned.

**3.** Add the olive oil. Then add sliced carrots and quartered mushrooms to the pot. Sauté for a few minutes until starting to brown lightly.

**4.** Add the seitan, cut into large, irregular cubes, about 1 to 1½ inches wide, to the pot, and mix well with the vegetables.

**5.** Sprinkle flour over the seitan-vegetable mixture and stir to coat well.

**6.** Pour the red wine into the pot. Add the fresh thyme, bay leaves, and salt and pepper to taste. Mix well.

**7.** Cover the pot with a lid. Let cook for 1 to 1 hour and 15 minutes, or until the vegetables are tender and the sauce has thickened.

**8.** Check the seasoning and adjust, if necessary, before serving.

## Tip

Serve the stew hot and with mashed potatoes, rice, or pasta, according to your preferences.

FOR 100 G

| protein: **6.7 g** | carbohydrates: **7 g** | lipids: **2.5 g** |
|---|---|---|

PER PORTION (350 G)

| protein: **23.5 g** | carbohydrates: **24.5 g** | lipids: **8.8 g** |
|---|---|---|

- FOR 3 PEOPLE
- PREP/COOK TIME: 30 MIN
- ALL SEASONS

# MAC NO' CHEESE SAUCE WITH CAULIFLOWER

10½ ounces (300 grams) **macaroni pasta** or **pasta of your choice**
3 cups (300 grams) **cauliflower**
4 cups (200 grams) **carrots**
½ (15-ounce) can (200 grams) **white beans**, drained and rinsed
2 tablespoons **nutritional yeast**
¼ cup (60 milliliters) **soy cooking cream**
2 tablespoons **cashew butter**
2 tablespoons **lemon juice**
1 teaspoon **Dijon mustard**
1 **clove garlic**, minced
**fresh parsley**
**salt** and **pepper**, to taste

**1.** Cook the pasta according to the instructions on the package. Drain, reserving 1 cup of pasta water, and set aside.

**2.** In a saucepan, bring water to a boil. Meanwhile, cut the cauliflower. Peel and dice the carrots. Add the cauliflower and carrots to the boiling water and cook until tender, 10 to 15 minutes.

**3.** Drain the cooked vegetables and transfer them to a blender. Add the drained white beans, nutritional yeast, soy cooking cream, cashew butter, lemon juice, Dijon mustard, minced garlic, salt, and pepper.

**4.** Blend until smooth and creamy. Taste and adjust the seasoning if necessary.

**5.** In the same pan, mix the cooked pasta and vegetable sauce. Use pasta water to thin the sauce if too thick. Heat over low heat for a few minutes, stirring, until the pasta is well coated in sauce.

**6.** Once ready, remove from heat, and serve the mac no' cheese garnished with chopped fresh parsley.

## Tips

- Use whole grain, bean, or lentil pasta for even more protein.
- You can make cashew "Parmesan" by mixing cashews, nutritional yeast, and coarse salt.

FOR 100 G

| protein: **7 g** | carbohydrates: **27.5 g** | lipids: **2.4 g** |
|---|---|---|

PER PORTION (350 G)

| protein: **24.5 g** | carbohydrates: **96.2 g** | lipids: **8.4 g** |
|---|---|---|

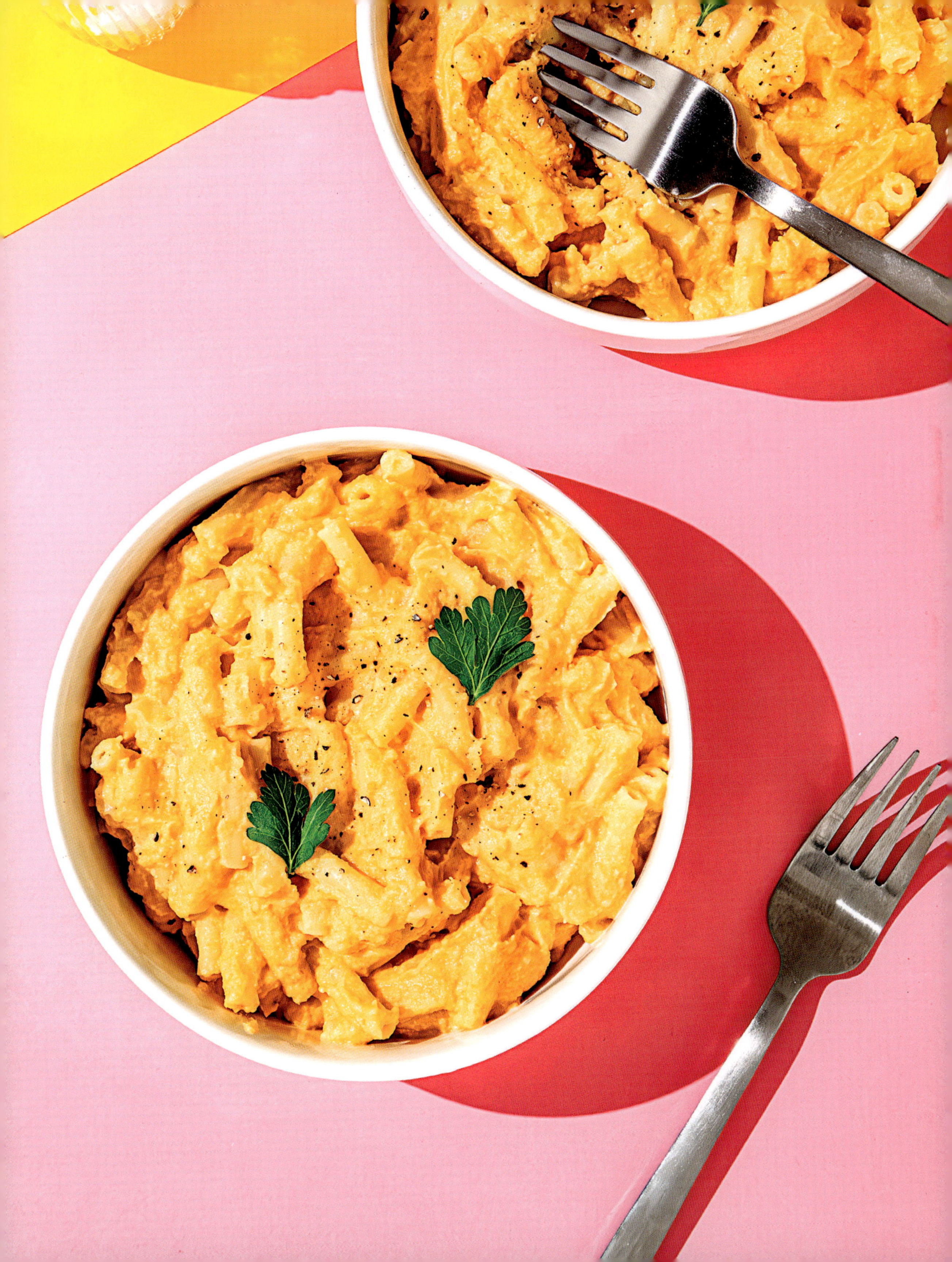

*Use these recipe cards to write down your own high-protein recipes.*

## RECIPE

Serving size: ______________

Prep/cook time: ______________

Title: ______________

Ingredients:

Directions:

## RECIPE

Serving size: ____________

Prep/cook time: __________

Title: ______________________________

Ingredients:

Directions:

## RECIPE

Serving size: ______________

Prep/cook time: ______________

Title: ______________________________

Ingredients:

Directions:

## RECIPE

Serving size: ____________

Prep/cook time: ____________

Title: ____________________________

Ingredients:

Directions:

# INDEX